FISH OIL
THE LIFE SAVER

FISH OIL
THE LIVE SAVER

Dr Caroline M. Shreeve
M.B., B.S.(Lond.); L.R.C.P., M.R.C.S.(Eng.); M.N.C.P.

Thorsons
An Imprint of HarperCollins*Publishers*

Thorsons
An Imprint of HarperCollins*Publishers*
77–85 Fulham Palace Road,
Hammersmith, London W6 8JB

First published as *A Healthy Heart for Life* 1988
This revised and expanded edition 1992
1 3 5 7 9 10 8 6 4 2

A catalogue record for this book
is available from the British Library

ISBN 0 7225 2487 0

Typeset by Harper Phototypesetters Limited,
Northampton, England
Printed in Great Britain by HarperCollinsManufacturing, Glasgow

For Janet Gale
with love

About the author

Caroline Shreeve is a qualified doctor with a strong interest in complementary medicine and how it can be married effectively with conventional medicine. She studied medicine in Dublin and London, has held several London hospital posts and was a principal partner in a general medical practice. She is now a freelance medical journalist and author of many books. Her chief writing interests are in the areas of women's health, emotional problems and the use of dietary supplements in achieving optimum health. She lives in Sussex.

Contents

Note to readers

Before following the self-help advice given in this book, readers are earnestly urged to give careful consideration to the nature of their particular health problem and to consult a competent physician if in any doubt. This book should not be regarded as a substitute for professional medical treatment and, while every care is taken to ensure the accuracy of the content, the author and the publishers cannot accept legal responsibility for any problem arising from experimentation with the methods described.

Introduction

The chance of writing this book presented an exciting challenge. As a doctor, I am well aware of the many thousands of lives claimed every year by heart disease. As an ordinary human being, which, after all, is what all health specialists are at heart, I know only too well how easy it is to postpone actually *doing* anything to minimize serious health risk factors until it is too late.

If you have not exercised properly for years, the undertaking to get fit may seem daunting. If you have eaten junk snacks and processed convenience foods all your life, the prospect of changing your diet is unlikely to appeal. Likewise, most people need to be strongly motivated to give up smoking and to learn and practise daily relaxation techniques. The vague concept of 'helping to ward off a heart attack' is rarely sufficient to tempt us to alter our lives in any radical way before disaster strikes. Yet the truth is we can do much – quite easily – to help ourselves towards healthy hearts.

One of the most exciting and important medical discoveries of this century is that a simple food substance which occurs naturally can minimize drastically the risks we all run of suffering from angina and heart attacks. Adding this nutrient to our diet on a daily basis offers extra protective action against cardiovascular problems. This simple means of caring for our hearts and arteries is available to all of us who wish to make use of it.

This is the story of the discovery of this powerful yet gentle supplement present in oily fish. Various aspects of this 'detective story' are outlined in the first five chapters, starting in Chapter 1 with a review of the problem of heart disease in Western society today, including the high-risk factors involved. Chapter 2 examines the fascinating epidemiological evidence leading to the discovery of fish oil's protective action. This evidence starts with the Eskimos' story, together with that of the intrepid explorers who journeyed far into the frozen wastes of Greenland to learn the truth about this race, among whom heart disease is practically unknown. It then continues with the Japanese story, showing that they, too, have a low incidence of coronary heart disease, particularly among those population groups who eat plenty of fish. The gradually mounting evidence of the protective action of oily fish is revealed, illustrated by an account of how the blood of Eskimos differs from ours and how an Eskimo diet altered the properties of the blood of a scientist who returned from Greenland and lived on an exclusively Eskimo diet in England for several months.

Attention then focuses on the famous 20-year study done at Leiden University. This examined the effects of eating fish upon the incidence of deaths from heart disease in a selected group of male volunteers in the town of Zutphen in Holland.

Chapter 3 bridges the gap between the mounting epidemiological evidence for the protective action of oily fish and the roles different types of fat play in our daily diet in the West. The meanings of terms such as saturated and unsaturated fats are given and the nature and importance of essential fatty acids, triglycerides, cholesterol and lipoprotein are explained.

Chapters 4 and 5 discuss atheroma and how its formation leads to atherosclerosis (furring up of the arteries) and the research that has been carried out into the safety and efficacy of fish oil in offering protection against this disease process.

The remaining five chapters present the Five-point Plan – comprehensive, practical advice on the steps necessary for keeping your heart healthy for life. Most people find it easier to make changes in their lifestyles if they are convinced that all the effort will prove worthwhile. Now pure fish oil concentrate has been shown to exert such a powerful protective action against angina and coronary thrombosis, as well as helping those people already suffering from heart disease, there seems far more point in making the required dietary changes, following exercise programmes, learning relaxation and giving up smoking, all of which will put you well on the way to a healthier life.

In conclusion, I should like to thank Seven Seas Health Care Ltd for the easy access they have given me to their research library and for the kindness of their scientific and technical advisers in answering my many questions.

Chapter 1

Heart disease – the risks

Throughout the ages, the main killer diseases have caused great fear in people. Before the advent of antibiotics, infectious illnesses inspired the most panic and horror and TB remained a serious problem until comparatively recently. Today, a diagnosis of cancer is the one most people dread beyond all others, even though approximately 50 per cent of all diagnosed cancer cases can now be cured.

Since 1981, the outbreak and spread of AIDS have caused alarm and anxiety on a colossal scale. There can be very few people who have not heard of its dangers and fear of catching it is having – and will continue to have – a profound effect on sexual mores until a cure is discovered.

Yet, despite all the panic and attention engendered by such diseases, there is one that is responsible for more deaths in this country than cancer or any other disorder, but which excites relatively little coverage. It is heart disease.

Facts and figures

In 1982, heart attacks killed 31 per cent of all the men who died in Britain, while cancer killed 24 per cent and strokes 9 per cent. The remaining 36 per cent were due to all other causes put together. Strokes, like heart attacks, are due to furred up arteries and between them these two disorders accounted for a staggering 40 per cent of all male deaths that year.

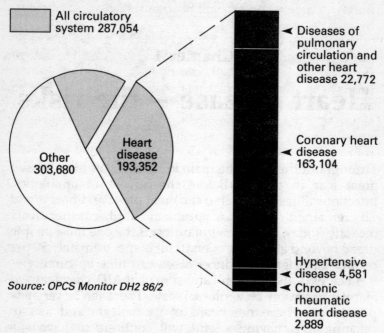

Source: OPCS Monitor DH2 86/2

Figure 1   Mortality in England and Wales in 1985

Deaths due to heart disease in women over the same period totalled 23 per cent and strokes 15 per cent, making clogged up arteries responsible for 38 per cent of female mortality. Cancer, by comparison, accounted for 21 per cent. Figure 1 shows the overall mortality from heart and arterial disease in England and Wales in 1985.

If we put the facts another way they make even greater impact: heart disease in Britain claims one life every 3 minutes, totalling 200,000 a year. One in five of all the men in the country below retiring age will have a heart attack before his sixty-fifth birthday, and one in two of these men will die. There are more deaths from heart attacks per head of population in Britain than anywhere else in the world, the worst 'death spots' being Scotland, Wales and Northern Ireland.

The problem in this country has been growing steadily more serious since the end of the Second World War. Over the last decade and a half, our death rate due to coronary thrombosis ('heart attack') has risen by 3 per cent in men and 10 per cent in women. Only in 1986 did it start to show signs of levelling off. Heart attacks were responsible for approximately 33 per cent of all deaths in Britain that year, representing a 3 per cent fall compared with 1985.

This is a hopeful sign, yet no reason for complacency. UK figures for 1989 shows that, of the 243,121 working days lost through ill health, 10.67 per cent were due to coronary heart disease (CHD) and an average of 5,817 NHS hospital beds are occupied each day with sufferers, costing £180 million yearly. The grim reality of heart disease is only just starting to make an impact upon British attitudes and lifestyles. Compared with the populations of countries with lifestyles similar to our own, we have a very long way to go. Over the past 15 years, the overall death rate from heart disease in the United States has fallen by 37 per cent, in Australia by 35 per cent, in New Zealand by 30 per cent and in Canada by 26 per cent.

Our attitude to health

There is a very good reason why Britain has retained the unenviable claim to the world's worst heart disease mortality figures. Compared to other nations, the British have remained impermeable to expert advice on minimizing the risk factors involved in cardiovascular disease. Other peoples have made radical and permanent changes in their diets, and have stopped smoking completely rather than half-heartedly 'trying to cut down'.

They have begun to counter stress by learning relaxation techniques and have taken up some form of aerobic exercise in the knowledge that their lives depended upon it.

The British, on the other hand, have chosen to turn a deaf ear to the repeated warnings of fitness experts and a blinkered – if not blind – eye to soaring cardiac fatality figures. Apart from the unfortunate few who are born with a defective heart or whose hearts become damaged by an illness, such as rheumatic fever, only a small minority pay much attention to the health of the circulatory system. Changes in lifestyles require effort and determination and for most people it seems it is easier to carry on doing what they are used to rather than face the facts and change.

This is particularly true in the case of diet. A typical example of a 'good old British standby meal' is fatty meat and overcooked vegetables plus greasy, thickened gravy and a pile of roast potatoes. Another is fatty chips with a hamburger or sausages, washed down by a pint of beer or an oversweetened canned drink.

In the UK people eat very little fresh fish, a surprising fact considering that the British Isles are surrounded by sea and the High Street fishmonger has sadly become a rarity. A recent survey among young, middle-aged and elderly people in Britain confirmed that the majority preferred fish prepacked and frozen, and preferably precrumbed and battered out of all recognition. The 'boil in the bag' sort, together with fish fingers, won hands down compared with fresh cod, plaice or haddock. A few middle-aged and elderly interviewees did bemoan the shortage of fresh fish and said that they would buy it more often if it were available. The majority of younger people said that they would not do so, as they had no idea how to prepare and cook it.

Our attitude as a nation to fish eating is more significant than it may appear on the surface. Not only has our consumption of fish overall in the UK declined, but our taste for fish has also altered. In place of the oily fish, such as mackerel, herring, sprats, whitebait, that were popular in Victorian England and the early part of the present century, we now choose non-oily varieties such as cod, whiting, haddock and plaice. These come from more distant waters, but have been made more available to us by the advent of freezer trawlers.

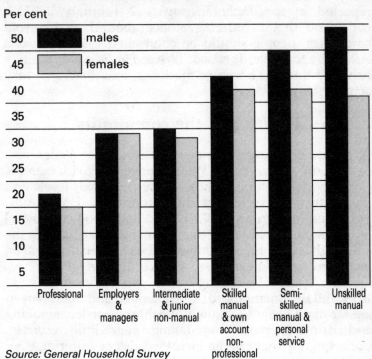

Source: General Household Survey

Figure 2   Cigarette smoking by sex and socio-economic group, Britain, 1984, percentages.

The figures provided in a report by the Ross Group, Grimsby, in 1980, show that the total landings of herrings in the UK in 1938 were 276,000 tonnes compared with only 5,000 tonnes in 1979. Over the same period, total fish landings fell from 1,121,000 to 929,000 tonnes, while cod and haddock landings fell from 513,000 to 243,000 tonnes.

Recent scientific research has revealed a vital connection between diet, especially the oily fish content, and freedom from heart and arterial disease. The report issued by the British Cardiac Society's working group (see page 29) was reported in the *Daily Telegraph*, 12 February 1987. It concluded that in offering advice about how to avoid coronaries, people should be counselled to eat fish as a substitute for meat. It stated: 'White fish is good, but oily fishes including herring, mackerel and sardines may actually be protective'.

Health and the community

A health organization known as Heartbeat Wales also carried out a survey in Wales during 1986 to examine coronary risk factors, high blood fat (i.e. lipid) levels and diet in various sectors of the community. The results, published in February 1987, showed that blood cholesterol levels are higher in Wales than in many other parts of the UK. High levels of blood cholesterol have been linked to an increased risk of heart disease since the early 1960s.

There is also a widening health gap between those in work and the unemployed. The unskilled and unemployed are far more likely to follow unhealthy lifestyles, smoking and drinking more but taking very little exercise. Consequently they run an increased risk of suffering from heart disease. Low-income families also eat more unhealthy foods, such as processed meat and fried meats, and buy fewer fresh vegetables and little in the way of fibre-rich foods. The health of non-manual groups and professional workers, on the other hand, has improved a great deal.

The 'fitness freak' label

It is tempting to brand people who do care about their hearts and arteries as 'fitness freaks', thereby dispelling any sneaking doubts about our own entrenched habits. Consequently, it is frequently the detection of high blood pressure during a routine checkup or the onset of chest pain following unaccustomed exertion which triggers serious thought on the subject. The nature of circulatory disease itself is also partly responsible. The furring up of arteries is a silent process that affects every one of us from adolescence onwards, yet it produces no symptoms until it is significantly advanced.

In addition, the very fact that so many people die of heart trouble means that there is a temptation to be fatalistic about it. We all know at least one person who has suffered a fatal heart attack and there is a tendency to feel that a 'coronary' is 'bound to get me in the end'. Circulatory disturbances of some kind, together with putting on weight and suffering from arthritis and rheumatism, are regarded by many sufferers as an inevitable part of growing older. In fact, some people seem to half will cardiovascular disasters to strike by adopting the attitude: 'When I go, I only hope that a massive heart attack finishes me off quickly'.

Of course death in some form remains inevitable for us all and a quick, sudden end seems preferable to a prolonged terminal illness. Nevertheless, a heart attack, or coronary thrombosis to give it its correct medical name, is an undeniably tragic event when it ends a man's or woman's life prematurely – both for the individual's sake and for that of friends and family felt to mourn. It is equally tragic when a major heart attack, instead of killing its victim outright, causes severe and irreversible damage.

Atherosclerosis

The growing problem of heart disease has engrossed medical research workers for several decades. Most people in Britain are now aware that the basic problem in angina and heart attacks is furring up of the arteries, or atherosclerosis. This involves the formation of fatty areas or plaques (i.e. atheroma) in the walls of arteries with consequent narrowing (i.e. sclerosis) of their interior channels. This reduces the volume of blood they are able to transport to various organs, including the heart, just as furred up domestic water pipes carry far less water than newly installed ones. The type of heart disease we are talking about here is ischaemic heart disease, often referred to as IHD. 'Ischaemia' means a deficient blood supply and is the explanation for both the pain of angina and the death of heart muscle following a coronary thrombosis.

Atherosclerosis is not a modern problem, however, despite the fact that it is now appearing as a mass epidemic in Britain and other countries with comparable lifestyles. The antiquity of atherosclerosis has been established from studies of Egyptian mummies and Leonardo da Vinci provided one of the earliest written descriptions of diseased, thickened blood vessels in the sixteenth century. This was followed by attempts to relate signs of disease in the coronary arteries that supply the heart muscle to symptoms of disease, particularly those of angina pectoris.

The term 'atheroma', from the Greek word for porridge, was not used in relation to arterial disease until 1904, when Marchand coined the term 'atherosclerosis'. This disease name is often used synonymously with arteriosclerosis, but the latter is really an older and more general term for thickening and stiffening of the vessel wall, a process affecting arteries diffusely and involving little in the way of deposited fat.

Atheromatous areas, by contrast, contain a great deal of fat and tend to be focalized here and there in affected arteries. Those supplying the heart, the chest, abdomen and pelvis (aorta), the legs (iliac and femoral), and the brain (cerebral) are particularly likely to be involved.

The interrelation between coronary disease, heart muscle

damage, and signs and symptoms of heart disease was eventually established when pathology emerged as a separate discipline in the second half of the nineteenth century, but it was not until 1918 that Herrick's suggestion of a relationship between clinically diagnosable heart damage and atherosclerotic coronary artery disease gained acceptance.

This may seem strange to us in the 1990s, but it is worth remembering that, at the turn of the century, Sir William Osler, probably the most eminent physician of his time, had seen only a handful of cases of ischaemic heart disease throughout the whole course of his career.

Risk factors

The concept of risk factors for atherosclerosis generally, and for coronary heart disease especially, derives from epidemiological studies, that is, from observation of the causes and distribution of the disorder within different population groups. The value of any 'risk profile' obtained in this way is that it helps to identify high risk populations in which a reduction in risk factors can be attempted.

An indication that a particular sort of lifestyle or diet incurs a higher risk than others, though, does not mean that the mechanism relating cause and effect is understood – it does not even mean that there is a certain *direct* interaction between a particular characteristic and the presence of disease. But what a comprehensive risk factor profile does do is help research scientists to isolate potentially useful areas of investigation which may reveal how the disease originates.

Age
The furring up of arteries generally starts in adolescence, though it has been known to begin in childhood. So the risk we run of heart attack increases with age, regardless of sex. The reason for this is not yet clear, but it is probably related

closely to our duration of exposure to other risk factors, particularly raised blood pressure and a raised level of lipids (fats) in the blood.

Average blood pressure in the UK rises with age, mostly because of the type of lifestyle adopted. Epidemiological studies of teenagers have recently shown that some individuals within this age group have blood pressure readings and blood lipids at the level of the general adult population.

Sex
Men stand a greater risk than women of having a heart attack during their early and middle years. A survey carried out in 1986 showed the greatest discrepancy between the sexes for those aged 45 to 54. In this group, nearly four times as many men died of heart disease. For patients over 75, however, heart disease was one and a half times more common in women.

If you are female, your sex hormones afford you a degree of protection from coronary artery disease up to the time of the menopause. Even so, the annual mortality figures for women in the UK show that 1 in 4 now die from a heart attack, and approximately 7,000 of these deaths occur in women aged under 65 years. In 1985, 82,131 women were victims of a fatal heart attack, compared with 104,467 men. The myth that 'women rarely die from heart attacks' is rapidly being dispelled.

Your risk of having a coronary is also greater if you are taking the contraceptive Pill, especially if you are a smoker as well. If you have an increased risk in the first place due to family history (see page 28), your safest plan is to give up smoking (or, better still, not start in the first place) and to choose an alternative method of birth control.

Blood pressure
High blood pressure increases the rate at which arteries get furred up with fatty plaques. The risks posed by high blood

pressure or 'hypertension', especially in men and women over 45 years of age, are serious. Anyone with a systolic blood pressure (the higher of the two figures in a blood pressure reading) greater than 160mm mercury, or a diastolic blood pressure in excess of 95mm mercury, runs *five* times the risk of coronary heart disease compared with someone of the same age and sex but with normal blood pressure. The risks of suffering a stroke are also greatly increased when the blood pressure is raised.

Smoking
Smoking – cigarettes and, to a slightly lesser extent, cigars and pipes – greatly increases the risks of an early death from coronary heart disease. Between them, the inhaled chemicals narrow and damage the coronary arteries and smaller cardiac vessels, encourage clot formation by making the blood more sticky, lower protective high density cholesterol levels (see page 30), and reduce the blood's capacity to transport vital oxygen to the heart's tissues.

Several major studies have been carried out to determine the extent of the risk and to highlight the age groups particularly affected. One involving British doctors showed that men under the age of 45 who smoke 25 cigarettes a day or more, run 15 times the risk of a fatal heart attack compared with non-smokers. Those between the ages of 45 and 54 years run a three-fold risk, and those aged 55 to 64 years run twice the risk.

Once you stop smoking, however, your risk of a heart attack decreases steadily and, after two years, it is no greater than that of someone who has never smoked.

Being overweight
Weighing more than you ought to for your height, sex and build increases your risk of coronary heart disease, and this increase becomes significant if you are 20 per cent or more above your ideal weight. Other risk factors that are especially likely to apply to you if you are too fat are high

blood pressure, a raised blood fat level (see page 30) and diabetes.

Diabetes

Diabetics, especially those who require insulin injections, run an increased risk of furred up coronary arteries and therefore of suffering from ischaemic heart disorders. The excess risk associated with intolerance of glucose, that is, with a raised level of glucose in the blood, can reach 100 per cent. This risk is slightly greater in women. It has also been found that, when a high blood glucose level is found in combination with a high level of blood fats, the total effect is greater than the sum of the effects of these two risk factors taken individually. This sort of action is called 'synergistic'.

Lack of exercise

Regular exercise has been found to decrease the risk of heart attack by more than 50 per cent, although the exercise has to be 'aerobic' – that is, it has to be sufficiently vigorous to increase the body's need for oxygen. (The value of exercise is dealt with more fully in Chapter 7.)

It is worth mentioning here the results of one study that examined the relationship between non-sedentary occupations and heart attack risk. Although only heavy physical work, such as that done by agricultural labourers or dockers, was found to be associated with a reduced risk of fatal heart attack, the decreased risk within such groups of people was very striking.

Family history

The close relations of coronary thrombosis victims run an increased risk of suffering a coronary themselves. In fact, genetic factors are implicated in about half the deaths that occur in Britain every year due to heart attacks. On 12 February, 1987, the *Daily Telegraph* reported the findings of a recent study carried out by the British Cardiac Society, a group to which all the country's cardiologists belong. One of the recommendations of that study was that identifying family members who are known to run an increased heart attack risk should be a major part of a national strategy for tackling heart disease. This would enable those people most at risk of a coronary to be screened for high blood pressure and raised blood fats and offered appropriate advice and treatment. Professor Michael Oliver, of Edinburgh University, who headed the working party responsible for the report, said that to screen everyone in the country for high risk factors was as unfeasible as it would be uneconomic, costing as much as 100 million pounds. Even so, fewer than 5 per cent of the population in the UK are screened at present, compared with 46 per cent in the United States.

Leaving unidentified high risk patients without appropriate health counselling and therapy explains, according to Professor Oliver, how such epidemics of heart disease arise in a community. His team had traced the family of one man who had a heart attack when he was 44 years old. Of the 51 first cousins who were traced, 46 – all in their thirties – were badly affected.

Anyone who believes him or herself to be especially at risk ought to take particular care to minimize their exposure to all the known risk factors. Tendencies to develop hypertension, diabetes and high blood fat levels are inherited traits and regular checkups can be life-saving.

Apart from the genetic element in familial complaints, we are all likely to 'inherit' both the lifestyle, values and attitudes of our parents and older members of our families. And far from feeling 'doomed' because a parent or other close relative suffers from angina or has had a heart attack, there is every reason to feel thankful at a personal level that our attention has been drawn to the problem in time.

The benefits of giving up smoking, weight reduction, eating less fat and taking up regular exercise are soon felt, which means that we can significantly increase our chances of avoiding cardiac disorders despite a family history of them.

Personality factors

Personality factors hinge to a large degree on an individual's response to stress. Personality types are broadly classifiable into two main categories – 'Type A', being those who run an increased risk of suffering from heart or arterial disease, and 'Type B', who are significantly less likely to do so. Type A people show a strong competitive drive, a sense of ambition and enhanced aggression. They also have a persistent sense of time urgency and a need to be forever on the go, usually with too many tasks. They find it very difficult to relax, looking for perfection in themselves and others, and have a tendency to become irritated and impatient at slight setbacks.

People with a Type B personality are the reverse. They are relaxed, phlegmatic and rarely perfectionist.

Raised cholesterol (lipid) level

A raised blood cholesterol level, referred to as the 'serum cholesterol', is highlighted at the end of the risk factor list, because of its enormous and unique importance in the development of heart disease. Cholesterol is a major component of the atheromatous plaques found in clogged arteries and experts examining the parts it plays in health and disease are now strongly in favour of everyone from the age of 20 onwards having their cholesterol level measured *at least* once every three to five years.

This can be done in a hospital's outpatients department, your GP's surgery or simply and safely at home using the recently developed Chemcard Test Kit. This indicates the cholesterol level in the blood by means of a colour change on a chemically treated colour chart (full instructions are provided). A finger prick of blood is applied to the pad and, after three minutes, the top layer is peeled back. The pad's colour is then compared to the surrounding sample colours, each of which represents a range of blood cholesterol readings.

Testing is especially important for people with a family history of heart disease and for the one person in 500 who inherits a tendency to high cholesterol levels. Males with this condition (hypercholesterolaemia), are known to run eight to ten times the average risk of developing CHD. However, whatever the cause of a high reading, the chances of a heart attack can be considerably reduced if appropriate action is taken.

As a guideline, a reading below 200mg/dl (5.2mmol/l) is healthy; 200–250mg/dl (5.2mmol/l) is on the borderline of high, but can be reduced by simple dietary and lifestyle changes within six to eight weeks; while 250–300mg/dl and above (or 6.5–7.8mmol/l and above) is above the acceptable limit and requires both medical advice and treatment.

Summary
● Heart disease is a major killer.
● Diseased arteries = angina and heart attacks.
● The main risk factors are age, sex, blood pressure, smoking, being overweight, diabetes, lack of exercise, family history, personality factors and raised cholesterol level.
● Measuring blood cholesterol is important.

The diet controversy

Atheroma is linked to a high consumption of fats, especially of the saturated variety, and consequently with a high level of fat in the blood. Dietary fats and heart disease risk factors have been the subject of great controversy for several decades. When many of the early studies indicted saturated fats as largely responsible for clogged up arteries, nutritional experts at first advised us to choose polyunsaturated (largely plant-derived) oils and fats in preference.

This was the start of the 'butter versus margarine' war and the sales of vitamin-fortified margarines forged ahead. It was then discovered that excessive amounts of plant-derived polyunsaturated fats were almost as bad as a diet rich in cream, whole milk, butter and fatty meat. Consequently, no one quite knew where they stood in the argument.

For a long time a high intake of cholesterol was considered to be the major culprit. Our knowledge of fats and their role in the human body is increasing all the time, however, and dietary fats, including cholesterol, have been found to exist in several different forms, grouped according to whether they have a high or a low density. While the low density types are known to be harmful, the high density sort have been shown to exert a protective effect against the development of atheromatous plaques.

Unsaturated fats have also been looked at more closely and far more is known now about the biochemistry of polyunsaturated fatty acids (PUFAs). Some of these are essential to us and are therefore called 'essential fatty acids' or EFAs. The majority of the EFAs have beneficial effects upon us and one or two have a mixture of beneficial and injurious effects.

Nutritional experts still urge us to increase the ratio of polyunsaturated fats in our diet in relation to the saturated (mainly animal) variety and, just as important, to reduce our *total* fat consumption as well. This recommendation is an important part of the advice provided in the two British government reports, one done by the National Advisory Council on Nutrition Education (NACNE) and the other by the Committee on the Medical Aspects of Food Policy (COMA).

It is now possible to go a step further and identify particular groups of EFAs which should be included in the diet for the protection they offer against heart attacks.

This advice on diet will be discussed in further detail in later chapters, but it should be emphasized here that *everyone* stands to benefit from following such recommendations for changing their diet and not just the minority of individuals known to have a higher than normal risk of heart attack. The style of eating proposed is a great deal closer to that of our grandparents and great grandparents during the first four decades of this century, at a time when heart and arterial disease were relatively rare.

Chapter 2

Learning lessons from the Eskimos

The link between an increased risk of heart disease and high levels of cholesterol in the blood was established in the 1950s and the early 1960s. The relationship was re-examined many times in a number of communities and found to hold good more or less universally. As a result, various ways of reducing blood cholesterol levels were tried, both through the use of drugs and by dietary intervention.

As we saw in the previous chapter, attempts to do so using vegetable oil polyunsaturates in the diet were not a great success. The trials showed no great difference in the overall mortality and interest in cholesterol diminished for about 15 years. However, research results published in the early 1960s showed that the polyunsaturated fatty acids (PUFAs) in cod liver oil were roughly three times as effective as those in plant oils.

The Eskimo enigma

Blood cholesterol levels became topical again in the 1970s, with the publication of the findings of two Danish medical researchers, Drs Jorn Dyerberg and H. O. Bang, who were working in Holland at the Alberg Hospital. They were interested in Greenland Eskimos, whose traditional diet is largely carnivorous and who have the highest consumption of fat in the world. Despite their diet – sometimes called a cardiologist's nightmare – the Eskimos were found to be surprisingly free from heart and arterial disease and from other degenerative diseases common in developed countries, including cancer, diabetes, appendicitis, diverticulitis, ulcerative colitis, dental caries, gallstones, acne vulgaris, multiple sclerosis and rheumatoid arthritis.

During their studies, Dyerberg and Bang made the fascinating discovery that those Eskimos who emigrated from their native land to Eastern Canada and assumed a Western lifestyle lost this immunity to heart and other diseases. A Western lifestyle, especially a Western *diet*, made them just as susceptible to heart disease and other degenerative conditions as Western people and they developed the same degree of risk within just one generation.

Also called Inuits – meaning eaters of raw meat – the Greenland Eskimos live mainly upon the raw and cooked fat and flesh of seal and fish. They eat practically no raw fresh vegetables or fruit and very few complex carbohydrates, grains, seeds and nuts. Consequently, they consume little vitamin C and little fibre. On the other hand their intake of polyunsaturated fats of marine origin is very high.

The Eskimo lifestyle includes plenty of stress, although of a different kind from the type we experience in the West. Although they are free from the pressures of modern living as we know them, the Eskimos have to face problems of very severe weather conditions, regular periods of starvation and the dangers of hunting and killing their prey. Some are smokers and some are obese. Nevertheless, heart disease is so rare among them, that they do not even have a word for it in their language (but they have 42 *different* words for 'snow'!).

Drs Dyerberg and Bang decided to approach the heart disease problem from an entirely different angle. Instead of trying to determine why so many people living a Western lifestyle die from heart attacks, they searched for a reason why so few Eskimos die in this way – what possible protective mechanism could be operating in favour of the Greenland Eskimo communities. At first, a genetic mechanism was believed to account for the obvious immunity these people enjoy. This idea was dismissed when it was discovered that the Danes, who are of the same Mongolian stock as Greenland Eskimos, are ten times more likely than Eskimos to suffer from ischaemic heart disease.

The two Danish researchers decided to observe the Greenland Eskimos in their traditional environment before the opportunity disappeared forever, as so often happens when Western ideas and ways permeate an ethnic group who have hitherto retained their own cultural ideas, lifestyle and traditions. So they organized an expedition in conjunction with Dr Hugh Sinclair, a well-known British nutritionist and an authority on Eskimo nutrition in particular.

The group travelled in the winter of 1976 to an Eskimo colony in north-west Greenland. They collected specimens for later analysis, including both dietary items – fish, seal flesh, etc. – and a number of samples of the Eskimos' blood. They were especially interested in the latter's fat content and in its clotting properties, to see if these could throw light on the apparent enigma of the Eskimos' high fat intake and their relative freedom from heart attacks, angina and arterial diseases in general.

On analysis, two very special essential fatty acids, known for short as EPA and DHA, were found to be present in Eskimo blood (more will be said about these later). What must be mentioned here are the other unique aspects of the Eskimo blood which were discovered by the researchers. These came as a hugely exciting revelation to the painstaking researchers who had travelled so many miles in their quest.

One of these discoveries, which served as an important

clue in the puzzle, was that the blood of their Eskimo volunteers did not clot as easily as normal, 'normal' being taken as the average or 'norm' as seen in the vast majority of other human beings. This was found to be true when their skin was punctured, with bleeding continuing for about eight minutes instead of the average four to five minutes, and when specimens of their blood were examined in glass test tubes. The explanation was soon found to rest with the platelets (tiny, cell-like particles in blood that encourage clot formation), which were far less active in this capacity than usual.

The second discovery was a low blood level of 'whole fat' (triglyceride), despite the huge amount of fat the Eskimo diet contains. Total levels of cholesterol were the same as those in the West, but it was distributed in a far safer pattern. The overall impression – one that has been confirmed many times over by subsequent studies – was that biochemical factors in their blood, afforded Eskimos a considerable degree of protection against arterial and heart disease.

Dr Hugh Sinclair was very intrigued by the initial findings. Because facilities for carrying out certain investigations were so limited when travelling by dog-sledge, he decided that the only way to carry out experiments was to go on an Eskimo diet himself, with some volunteers, on his return to the UK. Such an experiment would have the added bonus of showing how a Westerner's blood would be affected by this way of eating, as well as showing whether the protection the Eskimos somehow possess could be conveyed to a non-Eskimo individual simply by eating the same foods. His findings are best illustrated by describing the very courageous experiment which he performed after his return from the Greenland expedition.

Fish Oil

Dr Sinclair's diet

It was March 1979 before a deep-frozen seal arrived at the Institute of Human Nutrition in Oxfordshire, where Dr Sinclair worked, and the experiment could begin. In the end he decided to undertake the diet alone in case it should prove harmful in any way to people unaccustomed to it. He lived for 100 days on nothing but marine animal food – seal, fish and shell fish – and water. All the food he ate was weighed and recorded. A team of experts carried out a wide variety of tests, including sophisticated measurements of short-lived cell regulators called prostaglandins, seminal fluid analysis and muscle biopsies (that is, the removal of tiny fragments of body muscle under anaesthetic for study in the laboratory).

The results were subsequently published and a paper entitled 'The Advantages and Disadvantages of an Eskimo Diet' summed up the most important findings. The venture was courageous not only because of the unpalatability of the diet and the extreme boredom it was likely to generate, but particularly because little was known about how a diet so high in fat and protein, and almost totally lacking vitamin C, would affect a Westerner.

There was also the risk of vitamin A (retinol) toxicity. The livers of certain marine mammals – including Greenland seals – contain vast quantities of this vitamin and effects can be highly toxic. Many unsuspecting hunters have killed polar bears and eaten their livers to their eternal regret.

During the experiment, Hugh Sinclair's body weight fell from 96kg (15 stone) to a plateau of about 84kg (13 stone 2lb) and the fat layer below his skin reduced in thickness. His bleeding time was prolonged even beyond the average 8 minutes of the Eskimos. He also suffered from nose bleeds for the first time and bruises appeared spontaneously without previous injury. The number of platelets in his blood also fell dramatically, and those that did remain became enlarged and distorted.

At the same time levels of certain essential fatty acids dropped drastically, while others rose. And at the end of the diet, the very low density fats in his blood were greatly reduced, as the Eskimos' had been. Similarly, the high density type increased in quantity. And Hugh Sinclair's blood cholesterol level rose – from 175mg/dl (4.55mmol/l) on a normal diet to 185mg/dl (4.81mmol/l) at the end of the Eskimo one.

Although the level of vitamin A (retinol) in the blood increased by a factor of four, no signs of vitamin A toxicity appeared. In addition, despite the vitamin C (ascorbic acid) falling to zero in Dr Sinclair's blood, no signs of scurvy – the vitamin C deficiency disease – appeared.

The Eskimos' protector

Dr Sinclair's experiment provided much useful information about the probable reason why Eskimos are so free from heart attacks and other circulatory problems. Since their diet contains only very small amounts of 'N6' fatty acids and far larger amounts of the 'N3' type (also known as Omega 6 and Omega 3 – more about these in the next chapter), their blood is less apt to clot than that of people of other races. Eskimos have often been noted to bleed excessively from war wounds and Hugh Sinclair had noted how common nose bleeds were when he worked with Eskimo communities earlier in his career after the Second World War.

While bleeding too long following an injury can be a nuisance or, in some instance, dangerous, the 'thinness' of Eskimo blood and its slowness in clotting makes Eskimos far less prone than other races to thrombosis. Exactly how thrombosis occurs and the part it plays in causing atheromatous plaques inside arteries, will be discussed in a later chapter.

Metabolic disturbances resulting from a Westerner changing to the Eskimos' way of eating included failure to manufacture certain prostaglandin chemicals, an absence of spermatozoa (sperm) from the seminal fluid while on the diet and the production of certain essential fatty acids in a harmful form. These caused a degree of toxicity to the muscles examined, but fortunately no symptoms or signs of heart function disturbance. (Marine animals and Eskimos adapt to the effects of this toxic substance, which explains why they remain unaffected by it.)

A further problem with the diet was the low level of vitamin E. The result of vitamin E deficiency meant that the marine oils were likely to undergo 'peroxidation', a process which renders them useless. To counteract this tendency (always greater in a warmer climate), Dr Sinclair took a vitamin E supplement.

Not only Eskimos

The Dyerberg, Bang and Sinclair expedition had far-reaching consequences that remain very important to us today. Not least, they helped to substantiate many of the theories and findings of the epidemiologists, who continued their observation of other races sharing with the Eskimos an exceptionally low death rate from coronary heart disease.

The Japanese, for example, have a far lower incidence of heart attacks than might be expected, considering that their lifestyle is becoming more and more Westernized. It is easier in some ways to draw a comparison between the Japanese and Western peoples for this reason. They, like the Eskimos, are great fish eaters, many favouring their fish raw in the form of beautifully presented sushi that can surprise Westerners when first dining at a Japanese restaurant.

The effect of this high fish consumption on their blood fats was originally described by W. Insull, Jnr, and his fellow workers in an article in the *Journal of Clinical Investigation* in 1969. This paper also mentions that about 10 per cent of the dietary fatty acids found in the Japanese volunteers were of the variety that could only have been derived from fish or fish-eating mammals. By contrast, only about 1 per cent of those found in the American subjects taking part in the trial were of this type.

Insull and his team examined the dietary fatty acid content of their trial subjects by analysing samples of the fat layer below their skin, the subcutaneous fat. This finding was an important addition to the accumulating information about races who eat a lot of fish and those who do not. It showed that the levels of certain vital body chemicals connected with the consumption of fatty acids differed markedly between the two.

In addition, Japan's heart attack mortality figures vary greatly from one area of the country to another. The lowest death rates are found among the inhabitants of Okinawa Island, where the people eat about twice as much fish as their compatriots on the mainland. A notable discrepancy was also discovered by Japanese research scientists in the heart attack mortality rates of two villages in Chiba Prefecture. One of these was a fishing village, where fish figured plentifully in the people's diet, and here the death rate was very low. The other was a farming one where the consumption of fish was only one-third of that of the fishermen, and the death rate in this village was much higher.

Japan and the secret of the sea

Japanese fishing communities eat about 250 grams of fish per head of population daily. People living in farming communities, by contrast, consume only about 90 grams of fish each day. This means that Japanese fisherfolk derive about 2.6 grams daily of the valuable essential fatty acid EPA from the fish they eat, compared with the rest of the – non-fishing – population who derive only 0.9 grams.

It is interesting to compare these values with the estimated values of EPA intake in the UK per capita, firstly in 1848 when they were around 1.7 grams and then in 1978 when they had fallen to 0.2 grams. (It is also worth noting that intakes of DHA for 1848 and 1978 were 1.2 grams and 0.2 grams respectively.)

As was the case with the Eskimos, the difference in dietary intake of EPA in the Japanese fishing and farming communities is reflected in the total fatty acid analysis of the two groups. In fishermen, EPA accounted for 3.8 per cent of the total fatty acids and DHA accounted for 7.1 per cent. Among the farming people, these levels were 2.3 per cent and 4.5 per cent respectively.

In addition, the Japanese research scientist, S. Kobayashi, and his team found that the blood of the fishing people was thinner and less sticky (viscous) than that of the farmers and that their platelets were less inclined to clump together (aggregate) and cause a clot to form. H. I. Kato and his co-workers documented the relative coronary heart disease record of indigenous Japanese and of Japanese migrants to Hawaii and the USA. As was the case with the Eskimos who emigrated to Canada, there was a progressive increase in heart attacks and angina among the migrants, indicating a gradual loss of their previous immunity.

Other geographical areas where heart attacks are relatively unusual are parts of the Mediterranean, Anatolia in Turkey, and parts of Alaska. In none of these regions are the standards of medicine particularly high, the level of overall stress outstandingly low, or the inhabitants what we in the West would call 'health conscious'. One factor they do share, however, is that they all include fish in their diets.

The EPA mystery

Dr Hugh Sinclair proved conclusively that diet can affect both the levels of fats in the blood and its tendency to clot. Even these facts, however, combined with Dyerberg's and Bang's discovery of EPA and DHA in their Eskimo blood samples, represented only a small part of the complete picture. The question was from where had these two essential fatty acids come? The Danish researchers eventually traced their source to the samples of Eskimo food they had brought back with them for analysis, discovering that these two EFAs were present in the oil of the fish a.nd the marine animals that form the staple part of the Eskimo diet.

The whole 'food chain' has now been identified and it is known that EPA and DHA are manufactured within the cells of plancton (algae), minute forms of life to be found in seas and oceans the world over. These particular plancton, known as phytoplancton, are eaten by small fish which are in turn eaten by larger ones and stored in concentrated form in their body oils. The larger fish are then eaten by Eskimos, either directly or by a seal or other marine mammal which the Eskimos hunt and devour.

The significance of this may seem clear to us now, with the benefit of hindsight, but it is essential to remember that the parts played by EPA in human metabolism were as yet unknown (DHA is important to the nervous system and brain rather than to the heart and arterial system, so most references will be to EPA from now on). The Eskimos' unique disease pattern was well established, as was their relative freedom from heart attacks and other forms of heart disease. Further pieces of this intriguing biochemical jigsaw, however, still need to be found.

At about this time, a group of research scientists at the Karolinska Institute in Sweden and a separate group working at the Wellcome Research Institute in the UK were studying prostaglandins. These hormone-like, cell-regulating substances are formed in the body from essential fatty acids. It was eventually demonstrated that EPA could be converted into prostaglandins called prostacyclins and thromboxanes which, between them, influence the activity of blood platelets. In fact, it was later discovered that EPA encourages the production of prostaglandins that help prevent platelets from clumping together and discourages those that trigger thrombosis.

Dyerberg and Bang concluded from these findings that EPA was somehow the substance in the Eskimos' diet responsible for their freedom from heart disease. It appeared to exert its protective mechanism successfully in the face of the various dietary factors which might be expected to cause coronary thrombosis. Many research studies have supported and extended this view, including work by Tom Sanders of Queen Elizabeth College, London, which demonstrated that dietary supplementation with EPA could change the profile of fats in the blood and the tissues.

Confirmatory studies

Tom Sanders and his co-worker, Farah Roshanai, compared the effects of linseed oil with those of a marine fish oil concentrate upon the blood fat levels of healthy volunteers. Linseed oil contains about 60 per cent alpha-linolenic acid, an essential fatty acid from which EPA can be made. The fish oil concentrate – MaxEPA – is rich in preformed EPA (yet low in the vitamins A and D, thereby ruling out the risk of vitamin A toxicity).

The results of this study were greatly in favour of MaxEPA. Linseed oil raised the blood levels of EPA only slightly compared to the fish oil concentrate – even at a daily dose of 5g. At a dose of 10g, MaxEPA (but not linseed oil) significantly reduced the levels of both triglycerides and cholesterol in the blood and, at 20g, increased the proportion of protective high density cholesterol. Other trials have confirmed these findings.

Even when taken in small quantities, MaxEPA alters the fatty constituents of platelets in a healthy way, increasing levels of EPA and reducing those of a sometimes harmful fatty acid called arachidonic acid. Dr Philip Needham, a medical scientist, spoke about this effect at the American Heart Association Forum in 1981 and his report explained at least in part why platelets are less inclined to form clots when EPA levels are high. He said, 'Arachidonic acid serves in the body as the raw material from which the hormone is made that stimulates platelets to stick together. Therefore, replacing arachidonic acid with EPA in the platelets will reduce the proportion of the hormone and prevent unwanted platelet stickiness.'

Eskimo diets provide the daily equivalent of about 40g of MaxEPA. This is of practical interest only to Eskimos, but it is possible to transfer the benefits they enjoy to the West by eating more oily fish.

Experimental diets with a high fish content have been designed and used on volunteers as an alternative to administering supplements of fish oil concentrate. Dr William Connor, Professor of Medicine at the University of Oregon's Clinical Nutrition Center, for instance, created a 10-day salmon diet. Salmon, used in this way as a rich source of EPA, lowered the blood cholesterol levels of healthy volunteers by up to 17 per cent and by as much as 67 per cent in the case of patients suffering from raised blood triglyceride levels. 'The greatest effect seems to be in patients with elevation of both blood cholesterol and triglyceride levels', Dr Connor reported. 'The higher these levels are when the fish program is started, usually the greater the fall.'

Drs Dyerberg and Bang confirmed Dr Connor's results. They placed volunteers on a diet consisting largely of mackerel and again observed significant reductions in blood cholesterol as well as reduced platelet stickiness.

If you don't like fish or don't want to eat it every day, then take a fish oil supplement. MaxEPA is expensive and so is mostly prescribed by doctors for patients with clinically raised levels of blood fats and others at risk from angina and heart attacks, but to show how taking it compares with eating fish, the healthy changes in the blood that can be expected from dining upon 100–140g of salmon, can be equalled by as little as 10g of MaxEPA (the names of other fish oil supplements are given on page 149).

Summary

- Eskimos eat a great deal of saturated animal fat, yet rarely suffer from heart disease.
- Their blood
  - takes longer to clot
  - contains less 'whole fat' (triglyceride)
  - has its cholesterol arranged more safely.
- Studies have shown that other fish-eating communities (such as Japan) enjoy a similar immunity to heart disease.
- Eating more fish or taking a fish oil supplement can confer similar benefits.

The Zutphen study

This study provides one of the most persuasive arguments in favour of the 'high fish intake/lower heart attack risk' advice. It was carried out over a period of 20 years, and involved 852 men between the ages of 40 and 59 in the old industrial town of Zutphen in the eastern part of the Netherlands. This Dutch population was of particular interest because about 20 per cent of middle-aged men in Zutphen did not consume any fish at all in 1960. Others ate between 1 and 307g of fish daily. The average fish intake of the trial participants came to 20g a day, with about two-thirds consisting of lean fish, such as plaice, cod, and the remainder of oily fish, such as herring and mackerel.

Dr Daan Kromhout and his colleagues, who organized the trial, set out to investigate the relationship between fish consumption and coronary heart disease. This stemmed from their interest in the proposition that Eskimos rarely suffer from heart disease on account of the large quantity of fish in their diet. Careful dietary histories of all the volunteers, with particular reference to their fish consumption, were taken at the start of the trial, which began in 1960. Both the participants and their wives were interviewed about the former's eating habits.

During the following 20 years, 78 of the men died from coronary heart disease. Analysis of the results showed that the heart disease deaths throughout this period were inversely proportional to fish consumption in 1960. It was also clear that the number of deaths were 50 per cent lower among those men who consumed at least 30 grams of fish daily than among those who did not eat fish at all.

The findings of the study were published as a paper entitled, 'The Inverse Relation Between Fish Consumption and 20-year Mortality From Coronary Heart Disease', in *The New England Journal Of Medicine* on 9 May, 1985. The paper concluded with a recommendation that one or two fish dishes a week should be included in the dietary guidelines for the prevention of coronary heart disease. There is little doubt that considerably more fish – of the oily variety – could be recommended beneficially. Unfortunately, this presents a serious problem for people who want the protection from heart attacks offered by oily fish, and yet do not like or are unable to eat fish. Clinical trials carried out to test a recently developed answer to this problem in the form of a pure fish oil supplement will be discussed in Chapter 5.

Chapter 3

Fats and oils – good or bad?

It seems paradoxical that, on the one hand, the advice is to cut down considerably on the amount of fat we eat while, on the other, it is recommended that we incorporate oily fish in our diets as often as possible! Clearly, fats exist in vastly different forms and have very different properties, with certain types being dangerous if taken in excess, while others provide an element of protection. For most of us, edible fats and oils are simply bottles and packets of butter, margarine, lard and sunflower oil, with particular qualities that fit them for their various cooking and spreading purposes. We must look at them more closely to understand why fish oil should be so different.

Fats and oils

Most of the fat derived from animals – butter, lard, dripping, for example – consists largely of the saturated type, although it contains a certain amount of the unsaturated variety as well. It is generally solid at room temperature, a fact few people need reminding of in cold weather when butter becomes hard to spread. Most of the oils derived from plants, such as peanut, safflower, sunflower seed, olive, nut oil, are liquid at room temperature and contain far more unsaturated fat than saturated.

Margarine is generally made from plant oils. In some ways it is healthier for us than butter and the soft varieties are easier to spread when the temperature falls. The manufacturing processes used to make plant oils into margarine, however, also rob them of a number of their healthy properties.

A certain amount of dietary fat is vital to us. It provides us with energy – more, in fact, at 9.5 calories per gram than either protein or carbohydrate which supply just over 4 calories per gram. And, as everyone knows, food fuel taken in excess of energy used in physical activity is stored in the form of a fat layer below the surface of the skin. Here, it represents a readily available source of fuel and insulates us from the cold. Inside, layers of fat surround delicate organs, acting as shock absorbers and buffering them against injury.

In addition to these functions, fat deposits store certain drugs and 'neutralize' some of the noxious chemical compounds we inadvertently take in, by keeping them away from the main bloodstream and protecting us from their toxic effects. Fats also provide us with a number of necessary dietary nutrients such as the fat-soluble vitamins A, D and E and the essential fatty acids. Fat, too, provides the starter substances from which numerous body chemicals are made, the prostaglandins being one example – these are hormone-like cell regulators with very brief lives. These vital compounds will be explained in more detail later.

Saturated and unsaturated fats

These two important terms are often bandied around by people who have no clear idea of what is meant by them. However, a full understanding of the difference between these two types of fat is an essential first step towards comprehending just how fish oil can cut down the risk of heart disease.

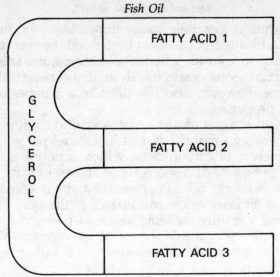

Figure 3 A triglyceride molecule

Most of the fats we eat exist in the form of edible oil molecules called triglycerides. The 'tri' part of the word refers to the three fatty acids which each triglyceride molecule contains, joined together by a 'bridge' called glycerol, which is another name for glycerine. The basic structure of a molecule is shown in Figure 3.

Fatty acids are the basic chemical building blocks from which oil and fats are made. There are some 12 to 15 different fatty acids present in edible fats and it is the variations in their properties that cause the fats containing them to vary as well. The fatty acid part of the molecule can be visualized very simply as a long chain of carbon atoms, linked one to another by chemical bonds like a string of pearls. Atoms of carbon have the capacity to link up or 'bond' with four other atoms. In a normal fatty acid chain one of those four bonds is used in linking it to its left-hand neighbour and another in linking to its right-hand neighbour. Each of the two remaining bonds are usually linked to hydrogen atoms. At one end of the chain, the last carbon atom makes up part of the acid section of the molecule (see Figure 4). When all the carbon links are occupied in this way, with none free, then the fatty acid is called *saturated* – that is, fully saturated with hydrogen atoms and incapable of attaching any more to itself.

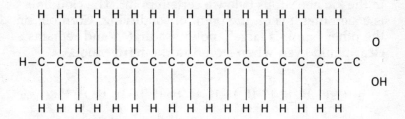

Figure 4   A saturated fatty acid molecule, typical of butter

Fatty acids can contain as few as 2 or as many as 26 carbon atoms. Normally, the 'row of pearls' contains between 14 and 22 carbon atoms, the commonest of all being 18. The fatty acid chain with 18 fully saturated carbon atoms is known as stearic acid and is commonly present in animal fats, such as butter, cream and lard.

Unsaturated fat is fat consisting of triglyceride molecules whose constituent fatty acids are not fully saturated with hydrogen atoms. Instead, two neighbouring carbon atoms are linked to one another by double bonds instead of by single ones. This means that, under certain conditions, more atoms of hydrogen could be added.

Fatty acids with two or more double bonds are known as *polyunsaturated*, simply meaning 'unsaturated in several places' along the carbon atom chain. They are often referred to as polyunsaturated fatty acids (PUFAs) and they contain among them those vital compounds the essential fatty acids (EFAs). PUFAs with 20 or 22 carbon atoms in their chains are called 'long chain' in order to distinguish them from those with 16 or 18 carbon atoms.

It is the state of unsaturation of plant oils that is linked to their liquid state at room temperature. Olive oil is an interesting illustration of this. The chief oil it contains is 'monounsaturated', meaning it has only one double bond in its carbon atom chain (see Figure 5). As most cooks who use it will know, olive oil goes cloudy when the temperature in the kitchen drops below a certain point. The cloudiness is a sign that it is on the point of solidifying. Corn oil, on the other hand, is largely polyunsaturated and remains a clear liquid even when stored in the refrigerator.

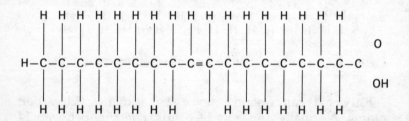

Figure 5   Oleic acid (18 carbons, 1 double bond), an unsaturated (or monounsaturated) fatty acid, typically found in olive oil

The position along the row of carbon atoms at which the double bonds occur in unsaturated fatty acids is crucial to many of their properties. It is usually described by numbering the carbon atoms from one end. Double bonds are not usually found before the third carbon atom on the chain, the fatty acids which have double bonds starting in this position are referred to as Omega 3 (N3) fatty acids (see Figure 6a).

Double bonds beginning on the fourth and fifth carbons are rare in biological systems. The next common place for double bonds to start is on the sixth carbon atom. Fatty acids of this type are referred to as Omega 6 (N6) fatty acids (see Figure 6b).

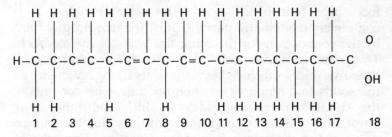

Figure 6a   Linolenic acid (18 carbons, 3 double bonds, Omega 3), an Omega 3 (N3) polyunsaturated fatty acid

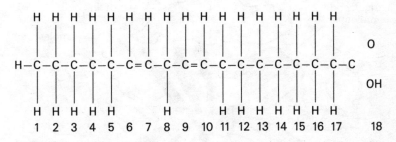

Figure 6b   Linoleic acid (18 carbons, 2 double bonds, Omega 6) an Omega 6 (N6) polyunsaturated fatty acid

The blood fats

'Lipids' is the correct chemical collective name for the triglyceride molecules and other fatty compounds within the bloodstream. The fats and oils we consume reach the circulation after the process of digestion has taken place. Perhaps the best way of grasping the idea of fatty acids and other essential fat compounds is to visualize exactly what happens to the fats consumed as part of our normal diet.

Solid fat, such as margarine and butter, is partly melted within the mouth as it is chewed together with other foods and warm saliva. It is then swallowed and passed down the food pipe (oesophagus) into the stomach. Here it is completely melted and partly emulsified into droplet form by the contractions of the muscular walls of the stomach. The stomach mixes solid foods with the mucus and digestive juices produced by cells of its lining, reducing all the solids to a liquid or semi-liquid state. The contents of the stomach then pass, little by little, into the small intestine, where they are mixed with and further broken down by the chemical action of the digestive juices formed by the pancreas and by cells lining the duodenum and jejunum.

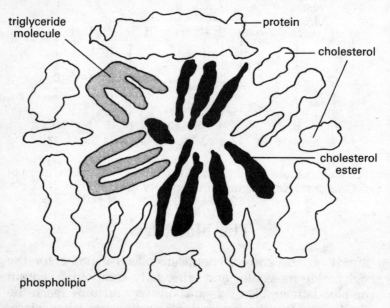

Figure 7 A lipoprotein ball in the blood (HDL type)

Lipase is the name of the organic catalyst or enzyme which helps to digest molecules of fats. It is produced by the pancreas and is responsible for breaking down the triglyceride molecules into their constituent fatty acid and glycerol fractions. This process, once believed to be complete, is now known to be only partial and much of the dietary fat is assimilated, unchanged, in the form of a very fine emulsion. This can only be produced provided there is enough lipase present to break down a proportion of the fat molecules, together with sufficient bile salts from the liver.

Once this part of the digestive process has taken place, the molecules of fatty acids, glycerol and unchanged triglyceride pass through the lining cells of the small intestine. Some of them enter the capillaries, the smallest blood vessels and thereby the portal bloodstream and the liver. Most of them go straight into the lacteals, the lymphatic vessels of the small intestine, and are conveyed by them straight into the main bloodstream, without passing through the liver first. Fat can then be stored or utilized at whichever points in the body it is most urgently required.

The lipoprotein

In addition to triglycerides, glycerol and free fatty acids, the lipid fraction of the blood includes cholesterol – a highly important fat – phospholipids, such as lecithin, and some hormones and vitamins. Being insoluble in water and therefore in blood plasma, lipids are able to remain suspended in the blood only after they have been formed into a fat/protein complex named 'lipoproteins'. The cells of the body carry this out by making an outer shell of water-soluble proteins, within which the triglycerides, cholesterol and other lipids are contained. These complexes take the shape of small balls (see Figure 7). The balls stay suspended in the blood plasma because of their water-soluble coating of protein. The percentage of proteins these lipoprotein balls contain ranges from 1 to 99 and determines their density and their size. The small, heavy, compressed balls are denser and more compact than the larger, lighter ones and are called high density or very high density lipoproteins (HDL or VHDL). They usually contain larger quantities of triglycerides and cholesterol and are heavier than water by between 6 and 28 per cent.

The less dense ones are low density or very low density lipoproteins (LDL or VLDL). They are lighter than water and contain far less lipid material and more protein.

The importance of HDL and LDL cholesterol

Cholesterol is often named as a major risk factor in cardiovascular disease, yet it has many beneficial uses in the body too. These include the manufacture of steroid hormones and bile salts and the synthesis of cell membranes. We obtain the cholesterol we need both from dietary sources and from our ability to manufacture it for ourselves.

The high density and low density lipoproteins between them transport more than 90 per cent of the cholesterol in the plasma of the blood. The beneficial or adverse effects of cholesterol depend upon whether it is incorporated within high density lipoproteins or within low density ones. The concentration of LDL cholesterol is directly related to the risk of coronary heart disease. The measurement of serum cholesterol in the blood – a standard test carried out as a part of a general health check and in people who are at a high risk of developing heart disease – reflects the LDL level. This has proved an accurate way of predicting the risks of angina and heart attacks over a wide age range.

HDL cholesterol levels are even more strongly predictive of the risk of suffering from diseased coronary arteries; but the levels of this sort of cholesterol have been found in nearly all clinical studies to be indirectly related to the risk. That is to say that, the higher the level of high density lipoprotein in an individual's blood, the *lower* his or her risk of heart disease. HDL has been known to exert a protective effect against heart attack deaths for a long time.

Much research has been aimed at discovering how the two classes of lipoproteins influence the development of atherosclerosis and clot formation (thrombosis). It is known that damage to the endothelial lining of arteries greatly encourages the entry of LDL from the plasma and the start or the further development of an atheromatous plaque. We will have more to say about the interplay of LDL cholesterol molecules and arterial disease in the next chapter. Regarding thrombosis, blood platelets show an increased tendency to clump together and set off the clotting process when in the presence of high concentrations of LDL cholesterol.

HDL cholesterol tends to be transported to the liver rather than to enter arterial linings and encourage atheroma to develop. This flow towards the liver even encourages cholesterol already incorporated within the arterial wall to be mobilized out of the early-forming atheromatous plaque – and elsewhere – and away to the liver as well. This is one of the ways in which HDL is believed to exert its protective action against coronary artery disease.

Another way is by reducing the uptake of LDL by cells – an essential prerequisite for atherosclerosis – by going into competition with LDL and getting accepted in place of it. HDL may also stimulate the release of a chemical compound, a prostacyclin, which itself has a protective effect against clot formation and arterial damage.

There are two other types of compound that are closely associated with our 'protection from heart attack' story which should be discussed in this chapter about fats and oils, these being the essential fatty acids and the prostaglandins.

Essential fatty acids

It is when we consider the fact that certain fatty acids are necessary to life and health that we start to realize not only that not all fat is bad for us, but also that some of it is very good indeed. Since we have seen that it is important to keep our total intake of fats under strict control, it is obviously crucial to pay attention to *which* fats we include in our diet.

Essential fatty acids (EFAs) are essential dietary components because they are needed for a wide number of metabolic functions and because the body is unable to make them for itself. Three such EFAs which have been identified are named arachidonic, cis-linoleic and alpha-linolenic acid, also known collectively as vitamin F. The first two are N6 EFAs, and the last mentioned belongs to the N3 class (N6 and N3 are the same as W6 and W3).

This is what Professor David Horrobin, international expert on essential fatty acids and prostaglandin chemistry, has to say about our need for the EFAs in his book, *Clinical Uses of Essential Fatty Acids*:

Medical specialists and authoritative national and international committees have repeatedly urged patients to take 10 to 15 per cent of their total calorie intake in the form of EFAs. This is in contrast to the 1 per cent of total calorie intake which is adequate to support normal growth and development in young animals. Curiously, EFAs are the only nutrients which the medical profession consistently advises us to take in mega-doses [the RDAs or 'recommended daily amounts' of most vitamins are expressed in micrograms or milligrams]. These mega-doses have been found to have desirable effects in a variety of conditions, notably cardiovascular problems.

We require about 5-10 grams a day of linoleic acid. It is provided by plant oils, such as safflower, corn or sunflower oil, and most of us take it in ample quantities. No minimal daily allowance is normally given for arachidonic acid, although most of us derive a plentiful supply of it from such food as meat and dairy products and it is also present in shrimps, prawns and certain seaweeds. Animals and fish have been known for some time to require alpha-linolenic acid and recent research indicates that we need it too. It is found in green-leafed vegetables, linseed oil and soy oil.

One of the uses to which alpha-linolenic acid is put is the manufacture of the heart-protecting eicosapentaenoic acid, already referred to in its abbreviated form, EPA. This is the best point at which to take a look at what the essential fatty acids actually do once they are inside us. We can then understand the functions of EPA within context.

The EFAs – their uses

The EFAs share all the roles we have already discussed as belonging to fats generally. They are also vital constituents of the cell membranes of all the cells in the body. They play an important part in transporting fat in the bloodstream and they are the 'starter substances' (precursors) of the prostaglandins (see page 69).

Our bodies soon make a deficiency of EFAs known to us. Signs of an acute lack of them, such as may occur when growing animals are deprived of them totally, include eczema-like skin rashes, thickened coarse skin, hair loss, poor wound healing, failure of normal growth, and damaged cell membranes – for example, when the skin becomes permeable to water and large quantities of body fluid are lost through the skin.

A chronic shortage of EFAs can lead to a very wide range of metabolic problems. There is a strong tendency in humans to develop a functional EFA deficiency with age. This is because, although ample supplies of the three 'vitamin F' EFAs may continue to be achieved through our diet, we become less efficient at utilizing them, with the result that our cells fail to synthesize a number of compounds that are vital to our metabolism. This is one of the possible reasons for the risks of heart attacks and arterial problems increasing with age.

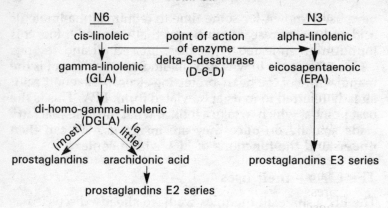

Figure 8   Metabolism of fatty acids and prostaglandins

The prostaglandins

An interesting fact about the three vitamin EFAs is that they only become useful to us metabolically once they have been transformed into something else! Their true potential lies in their being precursors, firstly of other EFAs and – ultimately – of prostaglandins. The process is carried out by the action of enzyme systems, an example of which is provided by the conversion of cis-linoleic acid into arachidonic acid. The carbon atom chain of cis-linoleic acid is elongated and further desaturated, in other words given more double bonds, with the result that the cis-linoleic acid becomes arachidonic acid.

Both of these EFAs belong to the N6 family, and this 'same family' rule always applies, meaning that N6 (starter) EFAs can only be converted into other N6 EFAs, N3 (starter) EFAs into other N3 EFAs, etc. These N6 and N3 EFAs are then converted into particular kinds of prostaglandins (PGs), for example, cis-linoleic acid gives rise to 1-series PGs, arachidonic acid to 2-series PGs, and alpha-linolenic acid to 3-series PGs. This lack of interchangeability between N3 and N6 EFA groups is extremely important. It means that it is vital to us that *both* types are supplied by our diet if we are to strike the right balance between the different types of PGs that we need.

The prostaglandins of the 3-series, into which alpha-linolenic acid and EPA are transformed, have as a group both similarities to and differences from those of the 2-series. They have both different and similar effects within the body. For example, the 3-series prostaglandins reduce the clotting tendency of the blood compared with PGs of the 2-series. In addition, high concentrations of 2-series prostaglandins are associated with heart disease, raised blood pressure and strokes. Prostaglandins of the 3-series block these harmful effects.

EPA derived from oily fish, if present in sufficient quantity, tips the prostaglandin balance in favour of the protective 3-series. For this reason, the ratio of N3 to N6 fatty acids in the blood is of prime importance. *This ratio is several 100 times higher in the Greenland Eskimo population than in the Western population.* The value of eating oily fish or taking a pure fish oil supplement should now be becoming clear.

Alpha-linolenic acid, the vitamin F essential fatty acid provided by green leafy vegetables, linseed oil, soy oil, etc., can be converted into EPA. Since we need EPA so badly for its protective activity against arterial disease, it might appear that we would do just as well to increase the quantity of green leafy vegetables in our diet as to eat fish. This is not in fact the case, because the enzyme necessary for transforming alpha-linolenic acid into EPA is frequently only weakly active and, in practice, little conversion into EPA takes place. Another factor affecting the efficiency of the conversion is the presence of a relatively large amount of cis-linoleic acid which seems to inhibit the process.

One – undesirable – consequence of our modern diets containing large quantities of PUFAs may be a deficiency of both the heart protector EPA and its longer chain cousin

DHA (docosahexaenoic acid) which plays a vital role in brain, nerve and eye tissue.

In the next chapter we will see how atheromatous plaques form in the first place and look at the way in which EPA protects the areas of metabolic function that other EFAs are unable to reach.

Chapter 4

How heart disease develops

The prevalence of atheroma in the Western world is almost universal. If you are a young adult – especially if you are male – it is likely that your arteries are already beginning to get clogged with atheromatous plaques which may eventually interfere with the flow of blood. You may look, and feel, fit and have no symptoms of any kind, but this very fact helps to underline the subtle nature of arterial and heart disease. It is a 'silent' process in the early stages and the time to start eliminating risk factors is right away!

The arteries

The easiest way to understand how atheroma affects arteries is to look first at where the arteries are situated, what they look like and what their function is.

Arteries are tubes of smooth muscle and elastic tissue which carry oxygenated blood from the heart and lungs all over the body. The largest artery in the body is called the aorta and its outline can be seen on an ordinary chest X-ray as it arches upwards and over from the heart's left lower chamber or ventricle. Other arteries branch off from the aorta and pass upwards in the chest and neck to supply the upper limbs, neck and head with blood. Then the aorta curves round and plunges downwards, running straight

Fish Oil

down in front of the spinal vertebrae or backbone, firstly inside the chest and then the abdomen, which it enters through a hole in the diaphragm. Throughout its course it branches off to the organs and tissues around it and it finally terminates within the pelvis in front of the fourth lumbar vertebra by dividing into right and left branches taking arterial blood to the lower limbs.

SMALL ARTERY

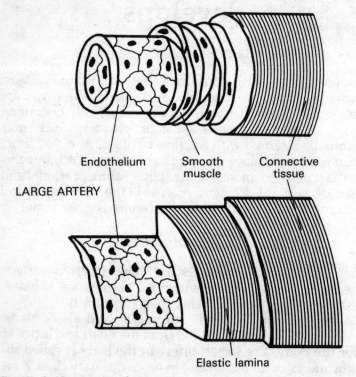

Endothelium   Smooth muscle   Connective tissue

LARGE ARTERY

Elastic lamina

Figure 9   Structure of arteries

Starting with the aorta, the largest artery, the arteries get progressively smaller as they branch away from the main arterial trunk, forming ultimately what is called the 'arterial tree'. Their internal structure is basically the same, regardless of their size, the main difference being that the larger arteries have more elastic connective tissue in their walls, while the smaller ones have a greater proportion of smooth muscle fibres (see Figure 9).

Atheroma

Despite the enormous amount of research that has been carried out into the nature and development of atheroma, this highly complex process is still imperfectly understood. Many tentative explanations have been put forward, but so far there has been no single, unifying theory capable of relating all the risk factors with all the possible mechanisms involved. For that reason, the account given here is partial, provisional and simplified.

There are two main kinds of atherosclerosis, the *fatty streak* and the *fibrous plaque*. The problem begins in childhood, soon after birth. During the first ten years of life, the lining of blood vessels thickens and small, bumpy cushions develop where arteries branch. This thickening affects all population groups so far studied, but it is especially prominent among races of people with a high mortality rate from heart disease.

Fatty streaks

Fatty streaks also appear in people of all races. They develop from collections of fats in the thickened arterial lining. These soft, yellow bumps appear in the walls of arteries, reaching a peak in size and number in people aged 20 to 30 years. One idea put forward to explain this phenomenon, based on studies of animals on high-fat diets, makes the following suggestion: white blood cells, called monocytes, stick to the flat, plate-like (endothelial) cells lining the arteries, push their way between them, then transform into scavenger cells called macrophages, capable

of engulfing other cells. They take in fat particles, becoming
known as 'foam cells' when they are full to completion. A
collection of these foam cells within the lining of the artery
constitutes a fatty streak.

Fibrous plaques

In people prone to atherosclerosis, fibrous plaques start to
appear after the age of 20 and become more numerous as
time passes, especially in common disease sites such as the
coronary arteries supplying the heart. Plaques develop in
the main from fatty streaks, although there is some
evidence that they can develop in areas where no fatty
streaks exist. The key event that prompts fatty streaks to
develop into fibrous plaques is believed to be some sort of
damage to the endothelial lining of the arteries concerned.

Experts who favour a haemodynamic explanation for
damaged arterial linings believe that in many cases the
injury is caused by blood flow turbulence. If one takes into
account the one and a half gallons of blood that get pumped
through the entire arterial tree every minute under
considerable pressure, it seems inevitable that the delicate
lining cells will eventually be damaged. This is thought to
be especially likely when blood pressure is raised, a theory
which goes some way to explaining the increased risk of
coronary thrombosis experienced by people suffering from
hypertension.

A large fatty streak may itself be the cause of plaque
formation, whether or not the lining has been damaged.
What is known for sure is that its presence in the arterial
lining triggers the blood platelets to clump together and
stick in a heap to the inside of the blood vessel. This
clumping action is very useful, since it forms the basis of
the blood clotting process that prevents us from bleeding
to death every time we cut ourselves. If you cut your finger,
for example, the platelets stick together and plug the gap
in the flesh and skin. The platelets release certain

chemicals, and fibrin threads are formed from the blood protein fibrinogen. These further block the gap by entangling red and white blood cells among them like fish in a net – the bleeding stops and repair work can start.

However, when all this takes place within the lining of an artery, powerful chemical counteracting activity (thrombolysis) has to be brought into play to 'switch off' the repair job. Otherwise the 'clot' or 'thrombus' plug gets bigger and bigger, playing a vital role in the formation of a fibrous plaque and eventually blocking the artery. Platelets repairing arterial damage release a prostaglandin named thromboxane, which has two main functions. One of these is to induce further clumping in the platelets which are joined by other blood cells, and the second is to constrict the edges of the breach in the damaged arterial wall, thereby narrowing it. These actions stimulate many of the cells in the area, especially the macrophages, into action and promote the absorption of lipoprotein balls into the developing plaque, together with their triglyceride and cholesterol content.

With repeated injury, the endothelial cell lining of the artery becomes further thickened and fibrous in consistency and tiny blood vessels (capillaries) burrow through from the outer layer of the arterial lining to supply the newly formed tissue. Sometimes either this blood supply is insufficient or a small haemorrhage occurs within the substance of the lesion. Its fibrous 'cap' then ruptures and releases a lump of fatty material into the bloodstream from the inside of the plaque. This is known as an embolus and it is dangerous because it can get caught in a small artery, so blocking the passage of blood within.

A question of balance

Clotting activity is normally kept within safe limits and thrombus, or clot formation, is avoided by a powerful prostaglandin called prostacycline, produced by the arteries. Often, though, the platelets' clot-forming action goes into overdrive and the counterbalancing action of prostacyclin is overpowered.

The effects of a number of the risk factors mentioned in Chapter 1 can be explained, at least partially, by the effect they have upon the blood's clotting activities. The emotional stress typical of the 'Type A' personality increases the output by the adrenal glands of the hormones adrenaline and noradrenaline. These prepare the person for the primitive 'fight or flight' reaction which would have been appropriate in times gone by when dangers were of a largely physical nature. Nowadays, especially in people who are ill-adapted to dealing with stress, emotional turmoil and fear are more likely to result from the daily wear and tear of modern life, rather than from something tangible. These reactions are generally repressed, so they continue to make the adrenal glands work overtime, secreting extra adrenaline and noradrenaline.

High blood levels of the two adrenal hormones increase the clotting tendency of the blood. The chemical stress of tobacco smoking, pollutants and 'free radicals' (unstable, highly reactive molecules or atoms which in some circumstances disrupt normal biochemical activity) in fried and roasted foods and in overused cooking oil are all believed to overexcite the body's defence system in the same way.

Thromboxane and prostacycline, like other prostaglandins, exist in the body for only a few minutes before being destroyed so we have to have plenty of raw material EFAs on hand to make further supplies.

This is a good point at which to turn to Figure 8 on page 60. This shows how the essential fatty acids are converted into further EFAs and ultimately into prostaglandins. The fate of the various dietary EFAs we take in is all important, since it is the final balance of PGs with which we end up that determines the level of risk we run of developing angina or having a heart attack.

Prostaglandins, our hearts and arteries

So far, we have not said a great deal about cis-linoleic acid other than that we need up to 10 grams of it daily, that most of us consume ample quantities of it in our everyday food and that it can be converted into arachidonic acid. This was mentioned as an example of the fact that N6 EFAs produce other N6 EFAs, and likewise N3 EFAs can only produce other N3 EFAs. Fortunately for us (and for guinea pigs who resemble us in this respect!), the conversion of DGLA into arachidonic acid takes place at a very slow rate indeed. Some experts even doubt whether it actually happens in human beings at all.

The reasons that it is fortunate have already been mentioned, but the different properties of the prostaglandins into which arachidonic acid can be changed, make it very much a mixed blessing. Prostacycline, known as PG12, is beneficial (besides discouraging clot formation, it relaxes the walls of arteries, helping the blood within to circulate freely), but two other PGs actually *trigger* thrombosis and encourage the arteries to go into spasm. Arachidonic acid also gives rise to leukotrienes – chemicals like prostaglandins that promote inflammation.

Considering arachidonic acid's bad points, our diets clearly provide us with more than enough of it since it is present in meat and dairy products. So two reasons can be seen for limiting the quantity we eat of these foods, firstly for their saturated fat content and secondly because of the arachidonic acid they contain.

The conversion pathway cis-linoleic acid normally takes is through gamma-linolenic acid (GLA) and DGLA to the highly desirable prostaglandins of the 1-series, which have very beneficial effects upon the heart and circulation. They lower the total amount of cholesterol in the blood by reducing the quantity of dangerous LDL type while leaving the HDL (protective) fraction unchanged. They also lower blood pressure, discourage platelets from clumping and help the blood to circulate freely by reversing arterial spasm and combating fibrous plaque development.

We have already seen, however, that large amounts of cis-linoleic acid in the diet can inhibit the conversion of alpha-linolenic acid into the highly valuable protective fatty acids EPA. For this reason, it is vital not to go overboard about PUFAs and take too much cis-linoleic acid to replace saturated fats. The whole emphasis of the advice about EFAs is upon balance, and upon quality rather than quantity. It is vital to keep up our intake of N3 EFAs so that 3-series prostaglandins are produced in adequate amounts.

Factors inhibiting EPA production

A number of other factors, besides cis-linoleic acid, reduce the production of EPA from alpha-linolenic acid through their adverse effects on the enzyme called delta-6-desaturase (D-6-D) that masterminds the necessary chemical conversion. Remember at this point, that the N6 and N3 series of EFAs compete with one another for their different stages of conversion and that unless they are taken in the diet in optimal proportions relative to one another, one of them will always gain supremacy, producing its own particular PGs at the expense of the others. When 2-series PGs predominate and we run short of the 3-series, our risks of suffering a heart attack escalate at once. Not without good reason is D-6-D referred to as the gate-keeper for both the N6 and the N3 series.

Examples of these factors include:

* saturated fats in the diet
* 'trans' fatty acids, formed by the processing of vegetable oils
* diabetes
* alcohol
* the ageing process
* adrenaline

- starvation (although a restricted calorie intake may increase enzyme activity threefold)
- a very low protein diet, although a very high protein diet helps to activate it
- a high blood sugar level
- oncogenic viruses (the type of viruses believed to be responsible for certain types of cancer)
- ionizing radiation.

EPA in the body

In view of all this interference with making EPA, a necessary prelude to manufacturing 3-series PGs, it is hardly surprising that simply increasing our intake of alpha-linolenic acid is an unsatisfactory solution. The beneficial effects of taking EPA in its naturally occurring form, though, have already been demonstrated by Dr Hugh Sinclair's experiment with the Eskimos' diet. Taking EPA directly enables 3-series PGs to be manufactured with impunity, since the 'problem point', involving the first conversion step dominated by D-6-D, is bypassed. The effects have been demonstrated many times over by other research scientists and doctors, both in the laboratory and in the form of clinical trials.

Here are the reasons why EPA offers such invaluable protection against heart attacks and arterial disease:

1. EPA encourages the production of 3-series PGs and, when these are produced freely, the overall effect of all prostaglandins present is that they are *less* likely to trigger thrombosis than when 2-series PGs predominate.

Both prostacycline and thromboxane are produced whichever PG series is made, but the thromboxane derived from EPA has a milder trigger effect upon platelet clumping than the one derived from arachidonic acid and 3-series prostacycline is better at *preventing* platelet clumping than the 2-series variety.

Fish Oil

2. EPA can reduce the levels of dangerous low density lipoproteins in the blood, thereby increasing the relative amount of the protective high density variety.

3. EPA can lower blood pressure.

4. EPA alters the activity of the monocytes which, as we saw earlier, adhere to the arterial lining and change into scavenging macrophages. The presence of EPA means that these no longer cause atheroma to build up.

Summary

- Atheroma – the fatty material which clogs arteries – affects practically everyone in Western society to a greater or lesser extent.
- It can develop from fatty streaks in the lining of arteries or from a plaque, or 'plate', of tough material attached to the arterial wall, consisting of clotted blood (thrombus) and fibrin formed by platelet action in an area of damage.
- Prostacycline (a prostaglandin), produced by arteries, discourages clot formation, but can be overpowered by high levels of stress hormones, toxins and free radicals (supercharged molecules).
- The fats and oils we eat, and the EFAs they contain, determine the quality and quantity of the prostaglandins we finally make. We need PGs of the 1-series (derived from cis-linoleic acid) and of the 3-series (derived from alpha-linolenic acid) to counteract the harmful effects of some of the 2-series type.
- Alpha-linolenic acid has to be turned into EPA before 3-series PGs can be made, and various factors interfere with this conversion.
- Taking EPA directly, overcomes this problem and offers protection against heart and arterial disease in important ways, such as, by discouraging clot formation, lowering blood pressure, reducing dangerous cholesterol levels and helping to prevent the development of fibrous plaques.

● Angina, heart attacks and sudden death from VF (ventricular fibrillation) are all possible consequences of clogged arteries.

Atheroma and coronary heart disease

The heart circulates blood through the body by the pump-like action of its muscular walls. This muscle, to function efficiently and survive, depends upon a continuous flow of blood. It receives its blood before any of the other organs of the body, via the three coronary arteries that leave the aorta at its base. These carry the blood to all the areas of the heart, dividing up within its substance into finer and finer vessels to form a complex network.

In coronary heart disease, the blood flow within the coronary arteries is interrupted in a number of ways, the most important being interference with the free flow of blood by atheromatous plaque formation and scar tissue. The three major consequences of coronary heart disease are angina pectoris, 'heart attack' and sudden death.

Angina

This is the intense, gripping pain experienced in the chest and sometimes extending to the neck and left arm when physical or emotional stress are severe. The pain is caused by the heart muscle (myocardium) being deprived of sufficient oxygen to meet its needs, due to an inadequate blood supply. When the extra demand upon the heart's capacity ceases, its need for extra oxygen also ceases and the pain goes away.

Case history
Thomas D., at 35 years of age, had never had a serious illness in his life. He was moderately overweight and smoked cigars occasionally. Never having married or learned to cook, he lived on take-away food, and ate

hamburgers and chips at least three times every week. Then he had a minor car accident, in which the driver of the other car involved became extremely angry, threatening to 'butcher' Thomas. Confronted by this, Thomas felt weak and shaky and noticed a gripping pain in the centre of his chest, which passed after about 10 minutes.

Two weeks later, he was out cycling in the country near his home and found that the chest pain returned as he was cycling up a steep hill. He also felt breathless and rather faint, so he took the next day off work and consulted his doctor. Thomas' blood pressure, which had not been taken for years, proved to be elevated at 180/105mm mercury.

Thomas was sent to the outpatients cardiology department for some tests, including an ECG and serum cholesterol levels which were found to be elevated. Angina pectoris was diagnosed and he was advised to lose 9.5kg (1½ stone) in weight, exercise in moderation and stop smoking. He was also given a diet sheet to follow and began to include fresh fruit and vegetables, wholewheat products in his diet, as well as oily fish at least twice a week. He felt better and fitter a year later than he had ever done as an adult.

'Unstable' angina

This is angina arising at rest or anginal pain of increasing frequency, duration and severity. Until recently, this was generally attributed to intermittent spasm of the coronary arteries, causing episodic reduction in blood flow. Now this condition is believed possibly to be due to recurrent thrombosis at the site of a ruptured fibrous plaque.

Acute myocardial infarction

This is the medical name for the acute and sudden death, or infarction, of an area of heart muscle. It is sometimes simply referred to as 'MI'. Sustained failure of blood supply to any tissue will cause irreversible tissue changes and, ultimately, death. When this happens to heart muscle, the normal pumping action of the heart is disrupted.

The outcome and prognosis following MI depends largely upon the area of myocardium involved. When this is large, the outlook is poor. When relatively small, the chances of recovery are excellent, scar tissue forming to strengthen the area of tissue destruction. In nearly all cases, severe narrowing of a major coronary vessel due to atherosclerosis is found and the eventual occlusion of the reduced channel may be due either to a tear in the arterial lining or to thrombosis.

Case history

Annie B. was 59 years old when she suffered her heart attack. She was 19kg (3 stone) overweight, smoked between 15 and 18 cigarettes daily, and had gone through the menopause 10 years previously. She never exercised, and did not believe in healthy eating, claiming all such advice was a lot of nonsense. She boasted about the large cooked breakfast she ate every morning, with plenty of fried bread cooked in bacon fat and slices of white pudding. She also had a stressful job as secretary to a workaholic, tyrannical boss who wanted her to retire.

For several months, Annie had felt a bit giddy and breathless when she climbed stairs and had tried, without success, to cut down her smoking. She also noticed a pain in her chest which seemed to go up into her throat and even into her lower jaw, when she ran to catch her bus.

Then, one Monday morning, as she was leaving for work, she received a telegram telling her she had won a six-figure sum on the football pools. She became intensely excited and rushed next door to tell her neighbour, only to collapse in the hallway with agonizing central chest pain. Her friend called an ambulance and Annie was taken to the nearest general hospital, still clutching her telegram.

Tests showed that Annie had had a myocardial infarction, doubtless brought on by intense emotional excitement, and that her coronary arteries were moderately to severely narrowed. Her blood pressure was 190/115mm mercury and her blood cholesterol level was seriously raised.

In hospital, she was kept on a strict diet, forbidden to smoke, and advised about her eating habits. She left hospital nearly 6kg (1 stone) lighter, bent on losing more weight and pleased that she had stopped smoking. Determined to live to enjoy her unexpected good fortune, Annie found altering her lifestyle, especially her diet, easier than she would have imagined.

Sudden death

This is the term applied to cases where a person, often in apparently good health, suddenly collapses with minimal, or no, warning symptoms. Post-mortem findings show that severe atherosclerosis of the coronary arteries is a far commoner cause than a coronary thrombosis (a clot in one of the coronary arteries). Often, there is evidence of more than 85 per cent severe narrowing of the coronary arteries. Death is usually the outcome of ventricular fibrillation, in which the large lower chambers of the heart (ventricles) cease to pump in an organized manner and are unable to maintain the circulation of blood around the body.

About 80 per cent of people to whom this happens have a recognized medical history of coronary heart disease, but for the remainder, sudden cardiac death is the first indication of heart disease.

Case history
Albert S. was 36 years old when he collapsed and died during a golf tournament. He had complained about chest pain on two or three occasions to his wife, but had refused to visit his GP. He was slim and fit-looking, a non-smoker and fairly health conscious, eating wholewheat bread and cereals, fresh fruit and vegetables and cutting down on salt and sugar. Warm croissants with unsalted butter and black

cherry jam, chunks of butter on his baked potatoes and lashings of double cream with his breakfast muesli were his only dietary weaknesses.

The post-mortem examination revealed that Albert's coronary arteries were nearly 90 per cent narrowed by atheromatous plaque. In addition, hypercholesterolaemia – high blood levels of cholesterol – was common in his family, and he had never bothered to have his level checked.

Besides being the prime cause of ischaemic heart disease, atheroma is also a prime cause of cerebral vascular disease – disease of the arteries supplying the brain. This links it with senility in the elderly and with strokes in middle-aged and elderly adults, especially women. High blood pressure is a high risk factor and is itself in part due to atherosclerosis. Strokes kill 70,000 people a year in the UK and incapacitate many others, causing brain damage, emotional and intellectual deterioration and paralysis.

Narrowing of the arteries supplying the lower limbs – called peripheral vascular disease – is also a major problem in the UK. Furred up, atheromatous arteries are the underlying cause and the health problems ensuing from this condition include chronic circulatory problems, intermittent claudication, which is when a person develops pain in the calf muscles on walking a certain distance, due to insufficient oxygenated blood reaching the region and, in severe cases, death (necrosis) of tissues deprived of an adequate blood supply, leading to gangrene.

Chapter 5

Fish oil – the life saver

A wealth of scientific literature, in the form of research papers, clinical study and letters to medical and scientific journals, backs up the findings of the pioneer workers so far discussed. The marine lipid concentrate MaxEPA has already been mentioned in the discussion of Dr Tom Sanders' trial (see page 44). This was the study in which the effects of linseed oil, rich in alpha-linolenic acid, were compared with those of supplying EPA directly.

Early research examining the effects of fish oil on metabolic processes used whole oily fish or an oil extract, such as cod liver oil, on their subjects. MaxEPA was developed by Stuart Reed at Seven Seas Health Care Ltd in response to scientists' need to verify the actual part played by fish oil in the prevention of heart disease. This was a pure fish oil concentrate in capsule form, refined and standardized so that research workers had a scientifically prepared substance of guaranteed purity and strength with which to carry out their investigations. It was essential for them to determine both the safety of using a pure fish oil supplement and its precise mode of action in human beings.

MaxEPA contains 30 per cent EFAs belonging to the N3 group – 18 per cent EPA and 12 per cent DHA. Produced from fish flesh instead of from fish liver, its vitamin A and

D content are practically nil, so using it incurs no risk of vitamin overdose or toxicity.

Having been found safe and effective, MaxEPA is now used world-wide. It was granted a product licence in 1987 in the UK for the treatment of high blood fat levels. And a further 120 clinical trials into its beneficial properties are currently in progress around the world. The American Medical Authority on heart disease also include the taking of fish oil as a safety precaution in the advice they give patients anxious to stay free from heart disease.

Animals, healthy human volunteer subjects and patients with cardiovascular disease have taken part in the numerous trials. The studies have explored the relationship between reduced heart attack risk and oily fish consumption from a number of angles.

To recap: the epidemiological surveys of the low-risk groups, such as the Greenland Eskimos and the Japanese, suggested that fish oil may hold the secret (epidemiology is the medical discipline that studies the distribution of diseases). Then came Dr Sinclair's diet experiment and Dyerberg's and Bang's explorations and deductions. These tied in with the observation that Western people were eating more animal meat, vegetable oils and saturated fats and far less oily fish than was once the case. At the same time their diet was virtually devoid of EPA and DHA and deaths from cardiovascular disease were escalating. The question forming in most research scientists' minds was whether a need exists to supplement the diet of Western populations with foods rich in these two nutrients. As usually happens, most of the early trials were carried out on laboratory animals.

Experimental work – animal studies

Animal studies are useful because they allow the safety of feeding experiments and other research to be carried out before being tried on humans and they provide a baseline

of criteria by which to judge the significance of these
human studies.

In 1977, D. P. Sen and his colleagues took a look at the
effect of sardine oil on the blood fat levels of rats. The rats
were biochemically 'challenged' by being fed daily doses of
cholesterol (to ensure that their fat consumption was very
high), and bile salts (to give the extra fat load every
opportunity to be digested and assimilated). The test diets
included both hydrogenated vegetable oil and varying
quantities of sardine oil, either crude or processed, or in the
form of whole sardines.

The diet contained between 10 and 15 per cent fat overall
and the various forms of it were adjusted so that the sardine
oil contributed between 2.5 and 10.2 per cent by weight.
After the groups had been tested for between 50 and 60
days, the trial was brought to a close. It was found that the
rats fed on either sardine oil or whole sardines had
significantly lower levels of cholesterol in their blood than
the others.

Another paper, published in the *American Journal of
Clinical Nutrition* in December, 1978, detailed a trial
involving dietary fish oil and baby pigs. The object had been
to examine the influence of dietary mackerel upon the
condition of their organs and their blood fat composition.
The research scientists, Dr A. Ruiter and colleagues, fed
groups of six young animals on diets supplemented either
by mackerel oil or by olive oil, each oil supplement making
up between 8 and 10 per cent by weight of the diet.

After four weeks, the research scientists found lower
blood levels of triglyceride fats in the pigs treated with
mackerel oil and evidence suggesting that vitamin E and/or
the trace element selenium was deficient in both groups.
The likelihood of this was confirmed by a calculation of the
pigs' intake of these two nutrients. Another research team,
headed by Dr G. E. Hornstra, also found signs of this
deficiency in laboratory rats fed supplementary cod liver
oil. These two papers both underline the fact, now well

established, that an adequate intake of vitamin E and selenium is especially important when extra dietary PUFAs are being taken.

Hornstra's team also showed that the blood of their rats who had received cod liver oil, had reduced levels of certain prostaglandins involved in the clotting process and so it was slower to clot when tested. In a further paper, they were able to confirm the anti-clotting properties of cod liver oil, which they put down to an inherent anti-clotting factor in the oil because they could find no evidence of increased production of PG1 3. This anti-clotting factor is now known to be the prostacycline produced as one of the prostaglandins from EPA, with the beneficial effect of discouraging the platelets from clumping (see previous chapter), and extra *is* produced when diets are supplemented with EPA.

A few years later in 1982, Dr A. vas Dias and colleagues published a 12-page paper in the journal *Atherosclerosis*. Summing up their research experience, they said that they had observed significant changes in the rabbits' blood platelets. Their tendency to clump and prompt clot formation under a variety of circumstances was considerably reduced in animals fed on diets enriched with 60 grams of MaxEPA fish oil concentrate per kilogram body weight, compared with those fed on diets supplemented by corn oil or coconut oil.

This change was accompanied by an increase in the platelets' EPA content which, before the experiment, had been around 1.3 per cent of the total fatty acids and after 60 days of feeding them the experimental diet, was 5.4 per cent. Other research workers (including Dr Tom Sanders and his team mentioned in Chapter 2), who have used either animals or human volunteers for their studies, have also discovered that platelets take up EPA from a fish oil-enriched diet.

Experimental work – human studies

One of the first human trials was carried out in 1978 by von Lossonczy and his team. Cistercian monks and nuns took part in a three-week cross-over dietary experiment. 'Crossover' means that the volunteers were divided into two groups, each receiving different diets which, halfway through, were 'crossed over' so that by the end of the trial all volunteers had been given both kinds of diet.

The diet, high in EPA, included a 200-gram daily portion of mackerel, containing 27 per cent lipids, including 8 grams of EPA. In the low EPA diet, the fish was replaced by 150 grams of cheese. Both items were included as part of a normal diet, although linoleic acid was restricted and a low-fat margarine used to bring the total fat consumption into a more usual range. After the three weeks on the high fish diet, their volunteers' cholesterol levels fell from an average 216mg per 100ml (5.6mmol/l) to an average of 197mg per 100ml (5.12mmol/l) and their triglyceride levels fell from 80.4mg per 100ml to 50.1mg per 100ml, while the protective high density lipoprotein (HDL) cholesterol rose from 55.2mg per 100ml (1.43mmol/l) to 58.9mg per 100ml (1.53mmol/l).

The blood fats of the volunteers showed levels of 5-6 per cent EPA (and 7-8 per cent DHA) after the fish period, but after three weeks on the cheese period, the levels had fallen to 1 per cent, similar to the starting level.

Mackerel, having a high oil content and being cheap, palatable and readily available, has been used in a number of other trials of fish oil effects. In March, 1980, the *Lancet* published a paper by Dr W. P. Siess and his team, who had carried out a study of how a mackerel diet affected various aspects of platelet function. The researchers fed volunteers for a week on a diet containing 500–800 grams of stewed or smoked mackerel daily, plus some carbohydrate in an unspecified form.

They found a marked decrease in platelet clumping and less thromboxane (the prostaglandin produced from arachidonic acid that prompts platelets to clump). They linked this with the dramatic change they found in the ratio of EPA to arachidonic acid in the platelet membranes, which rose from 1.0 to 25.5 before the high mackerel diet was started to 5.1 to 15.0 after six days.

The following year, another high fish intake trial was reported in the *Lancet*, this time examining the effects of an increase in dietary EPA on bleeding time, lipids and platelet clumping over an 11-week period. In this study, the protein content of the diet was only partly replaced by fish and the latter included salmon as well as mackerel. The 2 to 3 grams of EPA which the volunteers consumed daily resulted in increased levels of EPA in the platelet membranes, accompanied by a fall in the arachidonic acid content. Their bleeding time was significantly prolonged and platelet clumping reduced.

The same effects were observed by Dr S. H. Goodnight and his team, in volunteers whose dietary fats were derived mainly from salmon (about 450 grams a day) and salmon oil (between 60–90ml a day). The platelet membrane ratio of EPA to arachidonic acid in this case increased significantly from 0.005 to 0.3.

Research workers have, on the whole, been lucky in finding volunteers prepared to eat large quantities of fish for days on end. We can only suppose that they managed to contact fish lovers for whom eating 0.4 to 0.6kg of mackerel daily would be no hardship. Despite this, a number of the volunteers in some of the trials have found a high fish diet somewhat unpalatable. Certainly, if a tasteless, pure fish oil dietary supplement had not been created in capsule form to overcome the necessity for a hefty fish intake, large numbers of the population would be unable to take advantage of fish oil's protective action.

Another 1980 trial was aimed specifically at testing the effect of salmon oil upon blood fats, lipoproteins and 'triglyceride clearance' (the removal from the bloodstream of triglycerides after dietary fat or oil has been consumed).

This was reported in the *Transactions of the Association of American Physicians* that year and the team comprised two research workers in the USA – Drs W. E. Connor and W. W. Harris.

They fed their volunteer subjects for four weeks on salmon oil diets. These diets were designed so that they provided 40 per cent of their calories as fat. In the treatment diet, this fat was 17 per cent N3 fatty acids and 4 per cent N6 (see Figure 8, page 60). The control diet contained no N3 fatty acids, but 18 per cent of the N6 variety. Drs Connor and Harris found that, after four weeks on the salmon flesh/salmon oil diet, their subjects showed significantly lower levels of total cholesterol (155mg/100ml, or 4.0mmol/l, in contrast to 187mg/100ml, or 4.8mmol/l); serum triglycerides (45mg/100ml versus 76); very low density cholesterol (VLDL) (9mg/100ml [0.23mmol/l] versus 15 [0.39mmol/l]); and LDL cholesterol (105/100ml [2.73mmol/l] versus 124 [3.22mmol/l]).

The protective HDL levels were not significantly altered. The clearance of triglycerides following a 50 gram fat load was also much faster when the fat was salmon *oil* rather than a control *fat*. In addition, samples of blood took longer to clot and the platelet counts were reduced.

Besides the trial Dr Tom Sanders performed with his colleague Farah Roshanai, comparing the influence of alpha-linolenic acid and EPA on plasma lipids and on platelets (see Chapter 2), Tom Sanders performed a further one in co-operation with co-worker K. M. Younger. Together, they studied the effects of 5ml of linseed oil supplement four times a day for two weeks, upon platelets and plasma lipids. Their subjects were four vegans, whose diets did not contain N3 essential fatty acids, and five omnivores.

Vegans eat no animal products of any type whatever, they avoid anything in capsule form if gelatin has been included and some even refuse organically grown vegetables from soil treated with a blood extract or bonemeal. Omnivorous people eat anything and everything they fancy.

The linseed oil supplement, which contained 54 per cent alpha-linolenic acid, led to a very small increase in the proportion of EPA in platelet membranes and in plasma lipids of the omnivores and an even smaller increase in the vegans, whose diet is rich in cis-linoleic acid (we have already seen that relatively high quantities of cis-linoleic acid discourage the conversion of alpha-linolenic acid into EPA).

When the omnivorous volunteers were given supplementary MaxEPA, containing 18 per cent EPA, (5ml four times a day), there was a dramatic increase in the proportion of both EPA and DHA in plasma and platelets and a corresponding reduction in the proportion of arachidonic acid.

This shows quite clearly that the preformed dietary EPA and DHA are far more potent than their precursor alpha-linolenic acid in changing the proportions of N3 fatty acids in platelets and plasma.

Dr Sanders also found that triglyceride concentrations in the blood were reduced by the MaxEPA supplement and not by the linseed oil supplement.

In another trial conducted by Dr Sanders, this time with Drs M. Vickers and A. P. Haines, dietary EPA in the form of MaxEPA in a dose of 20ml daily for six weeks was again shown to increase the proportion of N3 fatty acids in platelet membranes. The secondary effects were a reduction in plasma triglycerides – by up to 75 per cent – and an increase in protective HDL cholesterol and bleeding time. All of these benefits disappeared after the MaxEPA was withdrawn.

Certain clotting factors and blood pressure, however, were also lowered, and remained low afterwards, suggesting a longer term protective effect. Other parameters – the platelet count, clot lysis (that is, destruction) time and levels of fibrinogen and other clotting factors – were unchanged, confirming the general safety of MaxEPA. Lowered blood pressure was also reported in the results of a clinical trial carried out by Dyerberg and consequently interest arose concerning the possibility of using fish oil extract to lower high blood pressure in hypertensive patients.

Studies involving patients

So far we have looked at trials which have examined the effects of fish oil supplements on various parameters in animals and normal volunteers. Many studies have also been performed involving patients with cardiovascular disease. One such one took place in 1986, and is itself an example of this interest in fish oil's blood pressure lowering capacity. It studied the effects of dietary supplementation with fish oil upon systolic blood pressure in patients suffering from mild 'essential hypertension' (the type of raised blood pressure that arises for no obvious reason, that is, it is not the result of circulatory or kidney disease or an adrenal gland growth, or phaeochromocytoma, which is thought to be due, in the early stages, to spasm of the tiny branches of the arterial tree, called arterioles.

Study with high blood pressure patients

A number of volunteers – 8 men and 8 women – took part in the 12-week study. All had a diastolic blood pressure (the lower of the two readings when blood pressure is measured) between 90 and 100mm mercury, and a systolic blood pressure below 200mm mercury. After a two-month run-in period, each received either 16.5 grams of MaxEPA or an olive oil placebo daily. The trial was organized as follows: the patients were randomly allotted to one or other of two groups; 'cross-over' occurred, so that all patients had first one type of oil and then the other; it was conducted in a 'double-blind' manner, with neither patients nor doctors knowing until the trial was over which patients had received olive oil placebo and which fish oil at any given moment.

The mean blood pressure of the patients before they were allotted to their two groups, was 160/94mm mercury. Following a course of the placebo, it was 161/94.5; and after MaxEPA treatment it had fallen to 151/92.5mm mercury. In a lying down position, the systolic blood pressure was lower after MaxEPA than after the olive oil placebo, by an average of 5.84 per cent; in a standing position, by a mean of 5.66 per cent. The lower average diastolic blood pressure (lower of the two readings) following MaxEPA was not statistically significant.

Of the 16 patients involved in the trial, 13 reported finding MaxEPA as acceptable, or more acceptable, than previous treatment they had received for high blood pressure. Although there is increasing evidence that treating mild hypertension reduces the risks of heart, kidney and brain disease, both doctors and patients are often reluctant to start on a long-term course of drugs. The conclusion drawn from the results by the three research doctors who organized the trial – Drs P. G. Norris, C. J. Jones and M. J. Weston – was that dietary supplementation with fish oil (MaxEPA) may provide 'a safe, more acceptable and natural treatment for patients with mild essential systolic hypertension.'

Study with ischaemic heart disease patients

A very interesting study was carried out in 1982 under the direction of Dr Reginald Saynor, MSc, Laboratory Director to the Sheffield Cardiothoracic Unit at the Northern General Hospital, Sheffield. His team included Drs D. Verel and T. Gillot, and their findings were published the following year. Their aim was to study the effect of MaxEPA on blood lipids, platelets, bleeding time and 'GTN' consumption in healthy volunteers and in patients suffering from ischaemic heart disease, that is, those patients with angina, high blood lipid levels and/or myocardial infarction. 'GTN' is glyceryl trinitrate. It is generally taken in the form of small white tablets which angina patients place under their tongue to relieve chest pain. Reduced consumption, of course, indicates fewer and less severe angina attacks.

As is usual with such a trial, a 'baseline' fasting blood sample was obtained immediately before the trial started to establish the 'norm' for all the subjects involved. All of the subjects took 10ml MaxEPA twice daily. No dietary modifications were attempted and blood samples were checked thereafter at monthly intervals for two years.

The results were impressively in favour of the use of MaxEPA. The blood triglyceride levels were significantly reduced by the end of the first month and these lowered levels were maintained throughout the study period. The decrease was more pronounced in subjects with initially high triglyceride values. Total blood cholesterol decreased in a significant way by the end of the two-year trial period, in subjects who started the trial within the normal range (it decreased, significantly, far earlier, in subjects who started the trial with raised cholesterol levels).

At six months, levels of the high risk factor VLDL and LDL were significantly lower than their pre-treatment values. The platelet count was considerably lower than pre-treatment counts for the first six months. Thereafter, it did not differ significantly from control levels.

GTN consumption at 9 months in 12 angina patients was significantly reduced. Their angina had improved considerably since starting to take MaxEPA regularly. Increased bleeding time was noted in a small, sub-sample group after 12 months, although this did not exceed normal limits. No change in bleeding time was observed after just 10ml of MaxEPA daily.

Another trial of MaxEPA in the treatment of patients with ischaemic heart disease, looked at the effects of fish oil upon platelet behaviour. It was carried out with the co-operation of 13 heart disease patients, and a paper relating the form of the trial and its results was published in the

Lancet in 1982. The patients took 20ml of MaxEPA daily for five weeks, their medication, diet and smoking habits remaining unchanged throughout the trial period. No patient's condition deteriorated during the study.

The results included a significantly prolonged platelet survival time, and this was attributed to the increased concentration of EPA within the platelet membrane. There was also a fall in the platelet count in the blood and this wsa believed to be due to fewer platelets being manufactured, because of the increase in their survival time. The levels of two of the most important blood clotting agents decreased significantly and the white cell count dropped very slightly. Another excellent piece of news was a significant rise in the level of protective HDL cholesterol, despite the fact that the total blood level of cholesterol did not alter.

I have quoted a fair number of clinical trials in this chapter. The reason is that they represent scientific and unarguable evidence in support of the use of a drug-free way of treating our most important cause of death in this country. It can sometimes be more fun to read anecdotal accounts about how Mr R. or Miss J. responded to a new wonder treatment and how it solved all his or her problems – including everything from a broken heart to ingrowing toenails and the menopause. However, while it is easier for a reader to relate to people with names and personal problems than it is to 'subjects', 'volunteers' or 'patients', such accounts are strictly anecdotal and they do not carry much weight at the end of the day in the truly scientific sense.

It seems – even when one has made a thorough study of a vast batch of clinical trials – almost incredible that a common or garden substance such as fish oil can offer protection from, and help to overcome, such momentous health problems as atheroma and ischaemic heart disease. Nevertheless, that is the truth of the matter and my feeling is that the more hard proof written and read about it, the

sooner people are going to sit up and take notice, and
actually *do* something about their own cardiovascular risk
factors.

Here, then, are the results of another trial of MaxEPA's
effect upon bleeding time, angina and blood fat levels in
both normal volunteers and patients suffering from
ischaemic heart disease (some of whom had already had
a myocardial infarction). There were 143 subjects in this
study, including 15 normal volunteers. All of them took
20ml of MaxEPA daily for 42 months in an 'open' trial,
meaning both volunteers and doctors knew that MaxEPA
was being administered and there was no 'double-blind'
element to it.

Also, in a second trial, 16 men who suffered from raised
blood levels of triglycerides, *were* involved in a double-
blind, cross-over trial in which they received either 10
capsules of MaxEPA or 10 containing a corn/olive oil
mixture daily for 8 weeks each. There was a four week
'wash-out' rest period in the interval between switching
from MaxEPA to placebo or vice versa.

In the open trial, the triglyceride levels fell significantly,
and were more pronounced in subjects with high pre-
treatment levels. Cholesterol levels fell significantly, too, in
subjects with raised levels beforehand. Protective HDL
cholesterol increased significantly after one month and
remained elevated. By six months, levels of the dangerous
VLDLs and LDLs were reduced.

Bleeding time was notably increased in a sub-sample
taking 20ml of MaxEPA daily for nine months. Again, no
difference was noted when only half this quantity was
taken.

GTN consumption by angina sufferers was markedly reduced
following MaxEPA supplementation at a rate of 20ml daily for
nine months.

In the double-blind study, MaxEPA resulted in a more
effective triglyceride lowering than vegetable oil. A
significant decrease in total cholesterol levels was observed

only after taking the MaxEPA supplement. Protective HDL levels rose significantly after both supplements, the increase being greater in the MaxEPA group. The research team, headed once again by Reginald Saynor and T. Gillott, concluded among other points at the end of the paper publishing this trial, that MaxEPA lowers total cholesterol levels in people suffering from abnormally high levels before treatment commences; that it raises the levels of protective HDL; and that it has a beneficial effect upon angina.

Study with peripheral vascular disease patients

Despite the numerous problems that atheroma can cause, we have dealt almost exclusively with ischaemic heart disease. I did, however, mention some of the effects of atheroma elsewhere than the coronary arteries, in particular peripheral vascular disease in the lower limbs and intermittent claudication. A very interesting trial into the effects of MaxEPA on patients with this condition was carried out by Drs B. E. Woodcock and E. Smith and their colleagues and the results published in a paper in the *British Medical Journal* in 1984.

The particular line of enquiry these research workers took was to examine the effects of supplementary EPA on the 'thickness' or turgidity (viscosity) of plasma, which is the fluid part of blood, and of 'whole' blood, that is, plasma plus blood cells. At the same time they investigated the effects upon plasma cholesterol and triglyceride concentrations and upon the various types of lipoproteins.

The study involved 19 patients with intermittent claudication who were given 20ml of either MaxEPA or a corn/olive oil mixture for seven weeks in a double-blind trial. Four patients in the MaxEPA group and two in the corn/olive oil group felt improved. No differences in whole blood viscosity between the two groups were observed at the commencement of the trial and the average value of blood viscosity throughout the entire group was significantly higher than it was for a group of normal control subjects. The mean plasma viscosity of the patients was also raised compared with normal subjects.

'Whole blood' viscosity was significantly reduced in the MaxEPA group *only*, but plasma viscosity was not affected by either treatment.

The average plasma triglyceride levels for both placebo oil and MaxEPA-treated groups were above the normal range to start off with. Only MaxEPA led to a significant reduction and most of this reduction occurred in the dangerous VLDL-triglyceride lipid fraction, a decrease in the protective HDL also contributing. No changes occurred in either the total plasma cholesterol or in the protective HDL cholesterol levels.

The scientists involved in this trial concluded from the results that the changes in viscosity and 'flow' of blood resulting from supplementary EPA are of potential therapeutic importance in established arterial disease. They were not able to conclude from this one trial precisely how beneficial such treatment might prove, but they recommended that further studies should be carried out to discover how MaxEPA reduces blood viscosity.

Chapter 6

A five-point plan

While clinical trials and research studies are very fulfilling academically if they extend our knowledge of disease and its causes, perhaps their most rewarding aspect is the practical application of the discoveries to which they lead. Their purpose, after all, even more than that of satisfying intellectual curiosity, is to benefit as many people as possible, as soon as possible. There is no doubt that the research that has shown the protective action of fish oils is among the most momentous and meaningful work that has ever been done to benefit mankind.

The five-point plan

The most encouraging news about heart and arterial disease is that we can now *do* something constructive to minimize the risks for ourselves and our families. The news is equally encouraging for anyone who has already had one or more heart attacks, or, in medical terminology, myocardial infarction, or who suffers from angina. A dietary supplement, similar to MaxEPA which is now only available on prescription, consisting of pure fish oils is now on the market. I shall have more to say about this in the final chapter.

Any supplement – to permit it to work as hard as it can

on our behalf – must be included within the scope of a properly structured health plan, which incorporates the correct diet, exercise, relaxation and recreation. Such a plan inevitably includes a complete range of dietary supplements that ensure we are taking all the vitamins, minerals, trace elements, amino acids and a few other miscellaneous nutrients that we need for the lives we need. Research has revealed which nutrients afford us most protection from atheroma and clogged arteries and it is wise to take most of these in supplementary form as well as eating those foods that supply them naturally. Our need for a complete and optimally balanced diet affording all the nutrients we require is proportional to the amount of stress – emotional as well as physical – we encounter in our daily lives and most of us need as much help as we can get in this direction.

There are five points to the new health plan:
1. diet
2. exercise
3. relaxation
4. giving up smoking
5. taking supplementary pure fish oil, which is the most important among a range of nutrients that offer protection from heart attacks and angina.

Diet

In an earlier chapter, attention was drawn to how much less fish is eaten in the UK nowadays than in times gone by, when heart disease was a rarity. Far less meat was eaten, too, during Queen Victoria's reign, as only wealthy people were able to afford it every day – and it was among the monied classes that the occasional heart attack happened – while the poor frequently went meatless from one year to the next. Angina and coronary thromboses among the poor were exceedingly unusual.

Fat consumption during the nineteenth century was also

considerably lower than it is now, while protein intake was roughly the same as it is today. Far more of the protein intake came from vegetable sources, since complex carbohydrates (see page 96) figured in a large way in the daily menu. This meant that people at this time consumed more fibre, too, as over-refined, processed convenience foods were unheard of.

The number of heart attacks have risen slowly since the beginning of this century. Our diet has altered radically, too, both in the type of protein we consume – most people eat meat in some form or another every day – and in our far higher intake of dairy produce. We eat a great deal more fat, especially the saturated type because of this, and our complex carbohydrate consumption has also declined steeply. Per head of population, we eat far less bread than was once the case, fewer grains and smaller quantities of fresh fruit and vegetables.

Consequently we consume far less fibre and a great deal more sugar. Both adults and children suffer more from obesity due to refined sugar products now than was the case 50 years ago, when sweets and chocolate were an occasional treat, not an everyday necessity. Processed foods fail to fill you like natural ones, because of their low fibre content, and many contain synthetic chemical additives that colour, flavour, emulsify, preserve and thicken them to suit the palates we have acquired. Taking all this into consideration, it is hardly surprising that people who insist on organically grown fresh products and 'whole', unrefined foods, are regarded as health freaks.

The diet recommended here is a wholefood one and the aims are to reduce the intake of fats, sugar and salt, to include plenty of complex carbohydrates (which supply fibre as well as nutrients and energy) and eliminate processed 'convenience' foods as far as possible. Eating only 'whole' foods that have had nothing added to them and nothing taken away can be less costly and is certainly more palatable than relying upon the five-minute roast dinner and trouble-free prepacked chicken pie, frozen and dehydrated varieties. Not only do the latter generally contain a wide range of synthetic additives, they are also sources of much 'hidden' fat, not to mention a high calorie count.

Research over several decades has also illustrated the benefits of including as much raw food in the diet as possible. Leslie and Susannah Kenton discuss many of the research findings in their best-selling book *Raw Energy* (Century, 1985), all of which point to the fact that the bodily systems seem to benefit from a high intake of raw vegetables and fruit – and their freshly squeezed juices – seeds, sprouting seeds, such as cress, beans, alfalfa and nuts. They quote from the work of Roger Williams, one of the most respected authorities on nutrition in the West, who maintains that 'cellular malnutrition is at the root of ten times the number of disease conditions as clinically defined deficiencies'. The diseases Williams is referring to include atherosclerosis – hardening of the arteries and coronary heart disease.

Having pointed out the harm a typical Western diet is doing to so many people, the Kentons say: 'The healing and health-promoting properties of uncooked foods have been demonstrated innumerable times in the biological clinics of Europe . . . Uncooked diets, coupled with other natural methods of healing, such as hydrotherapy and exercise, are used to treat all kinds of illness . . . heart and circulatory disease . . . Chlorophyll, it seems, has an impressive record in the treatment of heart disease, atherosclerosis . . .'

The important elements of a healthy diet

Carbohydrates
Foods containing complex carbohydrates, that is, starches and fibre, are filling but not fattening. Their bulk and their fibre content makes the stomach feel full, so reducing appetite, without adding a large number of calories to your

daily total. Bread and potatoes are the very things many dieters cut out as soon as they decide to lose weight, yet it is these foods and others like them that are a dieter's friends.

How many of us have gritted our teeth throughout a day at work or at home, or even through a restaurant meal or a party, sticking gallantly to lettuce leaves and mineral water while everyone else is eating and drinking their fill, only to go home and take a couple of Mars bars and a packet of chocolate biscuits to bed because we feel empty and miserable. Yet it has been demonstrated without doubt that obesity is a major risk factor in heart and arterial disease, which is why complex carbohydrates are even better 'best friends'.

Besides wholemeal bread and potatoes, carbohydrates of this type include other products made with wholemeal flour, such as biscuits, cakes and pasta, other root vegetables, grains such as brown rice, wheat, rye, millet, buckwheat (a seed that is treated as a grain), barley and maize or corn, pulses (fresh and dried peas, beans and lentils), seeds and nuts. Not to be forgotten are the 'pudding' crop vegetables such as tapioca, sago and semolina. Many of these foods are also rich in protein and provide vitamins, minerals and trace elements, too. They are all excellent sources of fibre, while nuts and seeds, as well as certain grains and vegetables, also provide fat, chiefly in the polyunsaturated form.

Wholemeal flour, incidentally, is produced by milling the whole wheat grain, including the outer husk or bran and the inner wheatgerm which provides calcium and iron, vitamins B and E and essential fatty acids (mainly linoleic). If wholemeal flour is described as 81 per cent, it is wholemeal flour from which some of the bran has been removed. This type of wholemeal flour is useful in helping you get used to eating brown bread, cakes and biscuits, etc, and is easier to use than 100 per cent wholemeal flour for certain 'light' recipes, such as sponge cake and choux pastry.

Complex carbohydrates are so-called because the sugars and starches they provide are in their natural, complex state, bound together with fibre and perhaps other ingredients such as protein and fat. Food of this type is 'complex' in comparison with the refined condition of white sugar, golden syrup and the white flour, glucose, etc., present in commercially prepared products. Most importantly, eating whole wheat and fresh and dried fruit will gradually wean you from any reliance you may now have upon the rapid boost to your blood sugar level obtained by eating confectionery and junk food snacks.

Stepping up your blood glucose level by eating such food may make you feel energetic for a little, but the pleasant effects are short-lived. Refined carbohydrates eaten in bulk like this make many people sleepy rather than energetic, and the peaking blood glucose level falls as soon as your insulin has driven the sugar free in your blood into the cells of the tissues. This can cause what is known as reactive hypoglycaemia or low blood sugar, the symptoms of which may include tachycardia (the medical term for quickened pulse), weakness, trembling, faintness, nausea and headaches. Having suddenly to produce a lot of insulin at once is fatiguing to the islet cells of the pancreas and this is believed to be one of the causes of non-insulin dependent diabetes, the type that occurs in middle life.

Snacks with high sugar contents are not a part of wholefood eating. However, many wholefood dishes are naturally sweet, relying upon the sugars present in fresh and dried fruit, vegetables such as carrots and parsnips, freshly squeezed juices and no-added-sugar jams and fruit purées, to satisfy the tastebuds. If extra sweetness is required honey, maple syrup, date syrup, carob (a naturally sweet alternative to cocoa, similar to it in appearance and flavour) or molasses or brown sugar can be used.

There is no official figure for the recommended daily intake of carbohydrates in this country, but most nutritional experts agree that between 60 and 70 per cent of a healthy adult's diet should consist of unrefined 'whole' carbohydrate.

Dietary fibre
This is derived from the cell walls of plants. The complex carbohydrates recommended above supply ample amounts of fibre. The simplest way of making certain your diet has enough fibre is to choose 'whole' brown flour products, brown rice, etc, in preference to their refined and denatured equivalent. A large salad daily, especially one containing some cold cooked grains, nuts and seeds, is another excellent source of fibre.

The recommended daily intake of fibre in the UK is between 25 and 30 grams. This may sound a lot, but there is no need to think in terms of doggedly spooning bran over everything you eat. Adding wheat bran is no longer thought of as the best way of obtaining dietary fibre, anyway, as a large quantity taken at once as a supplement (rather than that present in wholemeal flour) can bind the calcium in your blood with the phytic acid it contains, thereby robbing you of accessibility to this mineral.

Oat bran, either present in porridge or muesli or cooked dishes to which oats have been added as the staple part, do not have this effect upon calcium, so 'getting your oats' every day is in fact highly commendable, nutritionally speaking! Muesli supplies a fair amount of fibre, incidentally. Quaker's *Harvest Crunch* supplies 7 grams per 100 grams, and Weetabix's *Alpen* supplies 8.4 grams per 100 grams. Oatmeal also provides 7 grams per 100 grams, and other examples of fibre are:

● *Spinach* is 6.3 grams fibre per 100 grams. This makes spinach a very good source of fibre, as you have to cook at least 350 grams (12 oz) per person for a decent helping apiece, since it cooks down to practically nothing. Thus, 340 grams (¾lb) will provide you with more than half of your total daily requirement of fibre.

- *Celery* is 4.9 grams per 100 grams. Include celery in a salad or grate it into coleslaw, or eat it with cottage or other low-fat cheese instead of biscuits.
- *Coconut* is 13.5 grams per 100 grams. However, do not eat a bag of coconut ice – even the home-made sort – in order to obtain the benefit of the fibre!
- *Wholewheat flour* is 9.5 grams per 100 grams.
- *Wholewheat bread* is 8.5 grams per 100 grams.

The main varieties of fibre are cellulose, which is present in the husks of cereal crops, pectin, (found in most fruit), gums and lignin, provided by mature root vegetables, such as carrots, turnips, swedes and parsnips, and the outer leaves of cauliflowers and cabbage.

These different types of fibre have a number of useful effects in the body. Cellulose helps stimulate the bowel and keep the passage of motions regular, at the same time guarding against stagnating food debris and the flourishing of undesirable bowel bacteria at the expense of the helpful kinds. Pectin is soluble in water, but it remains undigested and softens stools by increasing their water content. Lignin helps to protect us from the formation of gallstones, because it binds with bile salts. Most important to our cardiovascular system, pectin also lowers the blood level of the dangerous lipoprotein fraction (LDL and VLDL) that play a major role in the formation of atheromatous fibrous plaques.

Overall, the fibre in our diet is believed to guard us against a number of disorders. Besides cancer of the large bowel, diabetes, diverticulitis, certain hernias, piles, obesity and peptic ulceration, these include – most importantly in this context – high blood pressure, varicose veins and atheroma.

Protein
The disadvantages of eating red meat have already been outlined, chiefly in terms of its saturated fat content. Even

if you cut all visible fat off your chops, steak or stewing steak, grill sausages and drain them on absorbent paper before eating them and avoid fat-laden pâté, salami and similar products, you are still taking in too much saturated animal fat if you eat meat every day. If you cannot do without meat, eat it as rarely as possible and try to choose liver, kidney, heart, brain and sweetbreads in preference to your usual favourite cuts. Poultry is better for you than red meat. It is less fatty than lamb or beef, for instance, and can be made more so if you do not eat the skin.

If you love fish and can buy it easily, you perhaps do not eat that much red meat anyway. When choosing fish, opt for the oily ones for their EPA action – mackerel, sprats, whitebait and herring are all easy to cook, while tinned salmon, tuna, sardines and anchovies can be found in any supermarket.

Do not forget eggs as a useful form of protein – excellent, from the nutritional viewpoint, if cooked and served without fat. Some authorities warn us about the cholesterol content of egg yolk and advise us to eat no more than three eggs weekly. However, opinion is divided on this subject.

Pulses, nuts, seeds and grains are excellent foods for a 'healthy heart'. Eaten in combination, they give you the full range of essential amino acids, just as 'first-class' protein in the form of red meat and fish does. Eating pulses with nuts or seeds is generally complementary in this way, as are pulses with grains, and grains with milk products. Sometimes complementary are beans, peas or lentils with milk products, or nuts and seeds with milk products. Combining nuts and seeds with grains can sometimes offer all the first-class protein you need.

The recommended daily intake of protein in the UK is 65-90 grams for men and 55-63 grams for women. Certain factors such as stress, infection and excessive heat can increase our needs.

Fat

A wholefood diet which limits the intake of red meat and dairy produce, while obtaining the majority of its protein from fish, poultry, game and combinations of vegetable foods, automatically reduces the intake of saturated fats. It also keeps the total fat intake at a far lower level than that of the 'average' person in the UK, who obtains 40 per cent of calories from fats and oils.

This is not the same thing as saying that the average diet in the UK contains 40 per cent of fat by weight. Fat delivers more than twice as much energy in the form of calories as does carbohydrate or protein, producing 9 calories per gram for their 4. This makes fats and oils far and away the most fattening foods we can eat. The reasons, therefore, for keeping consumption of them to a minimum are many.

There is no recommended daily intake of fats in the UK in terms of weight. However, some nutritional experts believe that, ideally, a healthy adult between the ages of 20 and 50 should reduce his or her intake to below 10 to 15 per cent. This would mean that fat supplied between 20 and 30 per cent of the total amount of energy.

The best sources of PUFAs are cold-pressed cooking oils, such as corn, safflower, soya bean and sunflower seed oil, and margarine made from these, though remember that margarine has the same calorific value as butter. Commercially processed oils that do not come into the 'cold-pressed category' contain those 'trans' versions of PUFAs already discussed. Look, too, for soft vegetable margarines whose labels actually mention that they contain cis-linoleic acid. One such brand is *Vitaquell* produced in West Germany, and available in many health food shops.

Do remember not to be too lavish with products containing linoleic acid. Although it is an EFA and one of the most healthful sources of fat in our diet, excessive amounts of it in proportion to the N3 EFAs, in particular alpha-linolenic acid, blocks the synthesis of the EPA we rely on for a healthy heart, so it is wise to keep its consumption on the low side. It is also vital that you maintain a daily intake of EPA in its natural form. You can do this either by eating 100-175 grams (4-6 oz) of oily fish daily or by taking pure fish oil as a supplement.

Vitamins, minerals, trace elements
These, as well as amino acids, are discussed in detail in the final chapter of the book, with special reference to those which have a protective action on the heart and arteries.

Eating for a healthy heart

Having looked at the foods we should avoid and those we should aim to include in our diets, here are some ideas for actual meals, aimed at translating the theoretical advice into a practical reality.

Breakfast
Most people like breakfasts that are easy to eat and quick to prepare. Muesli fits this bill to perfection. There are so many possible 'variations on a theme' that it should be possible to buy or to create a muesli to suit everybody's taste. The particular points in favour of this choice of breakfast are its high raw and high fibre content and the complex carbohydrates, proteins and PUFAs it provides in its grains, dried fruit and nuts. The slow release of its natural sugars during the course of the morning and the filling effects of its bulk should also prevent you from wanting to snack on doughnuts filled with 'shop' jam and synthetic cream mid morning.

Wheat flakes are present in many commercial mueslis, but if you make your own, try flaked millet, rolled oats and perhaps some barley flakes in addition to these. Fresh fruit is delicious added to the cereal ingredients and so are a number of tinned fruits, canned in their own juice without added sugar. For instance, try strawberries with enough of their juice to moisten the muesli, instead of skimmed milk.

The dried fruit you add can be chosen from sun-dried raisins, sultanas and blackcurrants or from dried apricots, peach or a 'fruit salad' mix, either as it is straight from the pack or rehydrated by soaking it in water or natural fruit juice. To muesli with any (or all!) of these ingredients, you can add extra wheatgerm, yoghurt – try the rich-tasting Greek variety – cow's or goat's milk or a little soured cream as a special treat.

Good breakfast choices in place of muesli include wholemeal bread, with plenty of whole grain included, rye bread or barley bread, spread lightly with low-fat soft cheese or margarine, honey, low-sugar jam or marmalade or Marmite. All these are high in fibre. If you have the time and inclination to cook, then eat a grilled simmered kipper, some smoked haddock or a fish cake made with salmon or tuna fish.

Recommended drinks include freshly squeezed fruit or vegetable juice, mineral water, weak unsweetened tea or decaffeinated coffee.

Lunch or evening meal
Try to make this meal a large, raw salad every day. Steer as far clear of limp lettuce leaves, overripe tomato and vinegared beetroot as you can. Boil grains or pulses in water to which you will have added some chicken or vegetable stock, herbs or spices for added flavour, drain them and make them – when cold – into a salad with sprouted seeds, such as mustard and cress, alfalfa, freshly prepared salad vegetables, grated root vegetables, parsnip and small white turnips are ideal – together with a few cold cooked vegetables left over from a previous meal.

Try a selection of vegetables with which you may not at present be familiar, such as avocado pear, baby sweetcorn, radicchio, raw spinach leaves, fennel, tinned artichoke hearts and raw mushrooms. Fresh fruit is delicious added to a primarily 'savoury' salad – fresh orange segments, for instance, are very pleasant with mild Spanish onion rings, black olives and freshly boiled or raw grated beetroot.

Nuts make a welcome, crunchy addition to large salads. Young walnut halves are delicious, as are unsalted cashews. For a dressing, try 2 tablespoons of cider vinegar with a tiny pinch of salt, a grinding of black pepper and a level teaspoon of clear honey, to which you can add any herbs – fresh or dried – that take your fancy. Garlic is claimed to be very good for the health of heart and arteries and this is an excellent excuse for including it in any and every dish imaginable, even if your friends and family do not like it! If you live near a convenient source, try adding a pinch of washed, finely chopped broom or hawthorn blossom, either to the salad as a whole or to your dressing. Both are reputed to offer some protection against the development of atheromatous plaques.

Good sources of protein to eat with your salad – if you want more than whatever is supplied by the grains, pulses and nuts you have included – are low-fat cheese, a hard-boiled egg or some cold fish. Try smoked mackerel, tinned salmon or tuna, smoked salmon if it is your birthday, or a tin of pilchards or sardines. Home-made wholewheat bread (unbuttered) is excellent with this.

Evening meal (or main midday meal)
It is a good idea to start every main meal with a small salad. There is plenty of evidence that a 'digestive leucocytosis' happens every time we eat cooked food. This involves the migration to the intestinal blood vessels of large numbers of white blood cells (leukocytes). Here, they gather at the cost of a certain amount of stress to our immune defence system, which is consequently weakened and less able to perform its job of protecting us from cancer and invading microbes. Eating a small salad before eating cooked food prevents this from happening. Leslie and Susannah Kenton discuss this phenomenon in their book *Raw Energy* (Century, 1985).

If you have not already eaten fish during the day (or even

if you have!) you might enjoy fish for your main, cooked meal. Avoid adding oil or fat if possible – you can grill most fish just as well by brushing it lightly with a little low-sodium salt and fresh lemon juice. Alternatively, cook it in very little skimmed milk or water on a plate over the vegetables you are cooking or put it in the oven with a tiny flake of margarine, three or four tomato slices, a squeeze of lime or orange juice and some fresh parsley, all wrapped in cooking foil.

Try to choose fish such as herring, mackerel or sprats. White fish as opposed to the oily variety are still a good choice – go for whiting, cod, plaice or fresh haddock. Good 'meat' alternatives include some sliced chicken breast, turkey, offal, game or eggs and, perhaps, some low-fat cheese.

Baked potatoes in their skins, with some plain yoghurt and perhaps a chopped up garlic clove if you adore garlic, are tasty accompaniments. Be sure to eat the skins of the potatoes as well for their vitamin and fibre content. Puréed or mashed vegetables make a pleasant change – carrots, parsnip, turnip and swede are all particularly good served this way. Brussels sprouts are also delicious, mashed finely with a little margarine and a good grinding of fresh nutmeg.

Round it all off with a light dessert, say some fresh or stewed fruit, sweetened with a little maple syrup or honey, or low-fat cheese and puffed rice biscuits (no added salt), or fruit or plain yoghurt, or water ice or ice cream made from natural ingredients.

Try the following recipes, too, for practical ideas for eating for a healthy heart.

Breakfast

Fish can be used in place of meat, with or without eggs, if you are a dedicated cooked breakfast eater. All these recipes are for two people.

Scrambled Kippers

1 medium kipper fillet
2 large, fresh eggs
a little skimmed milk
a little reduced-fat butter or margarine
salt and freshly ground black pepper
2 large slices granary bread, toasted and lightly buttered

1. Simmer the kipper in a little water until it is soft, then keep it warm while you prepare the rest of the dish.
2. Scramble the eggs with the milk and fat, adding a little salt and freshly ground black pepper if liked.
3. Flake the kipper fillet, removing any bones, then combine it with the eggs and serve on the toast.

Piquant Fish Cakes

These fish cakes make a tasty substitute for smoked bacon or ham. This recipe is also economical, making use of leftovers.

100g (4 oz) cooked or tinned fish
100g (4 oz) mashed potato
1 tbs low-fat butter or margarine, melted, or olive oil
1 small egg, beaten, or 1 tinned tomato, drained and mashed
Worcester sauce, to taste
wholewheat breadcrumbs (sufficient to coat)
olive or safflower oil, for grilling

1. Flake the fish and combine it with the potato and butter, margarine or oil, the beaten egg or tomato and add Worcester sauce to taste.
2. Shape the mixture into 4 small cakes and coat them with the breadcrumbs.
3. Brush the fish cakes with a little oil and grill them until they are golden brown. Eat them hot.

Grilled Bloaters

Bloaters are herrings partially cured by steeping them in salt and smoking them. They have a slightly stronger flavour than kippers and are healthy and delicious. The watercress gives the dish an interesting flavour contrast and takes away any tendency to greasiness.

1 medium bloater per person
a little oil
watercress (optional)

1. Brush the fish with a little vegetable oil and grill them until they turn pale brown.
2. Serve with watercress if using.

Lunch

Fish is an easy option whether you're snacking or eating a full meal.

Kipperfish Paste

An old family recipe, this paste can be served as an appetizer at a main meal, but is delicious on toast and in sandwiches. You can use smoked haddock or smoked cod in the same way, although they do contain less EPA.

1 large kipper
melted butter or margarine, to mix
freshly grated nutmeg and white pepper

1. Grill the kipper. Remove any bones when it has cooked and flake it into a bowl.
2. Mix the fish with enough melted butter or margarine to make a smooth paste.
3. Flavour the fishpaste with the spices and chill it well.

Tuna Alaska

Very few people would turn down tuna mixed with a good mayonnaise, sandwiched between slices of *fresh* white bread!

1×185g (6½ oz) tin of tuna
2 tbs mayonnaise made with olive or sunflower oil
4 slices, fresh white bread, buttered
2 spring onions, chopped (optional)

1. Drain the tuna, then flake it into a bowl and combine it thoroughly with the mayonnaise and spring onion, if using.
2. Spread the tuna mixture evenly on 2 slices of bread and top each with a second slice.

Salmon Brunch

This dish is simple and quick to prepare and makes an excellent light lunch or supper. Vegetables or rice served with it make a more substantial meal.

1×225g (8 oz) tin pink or red salmon, drained
1×100g (4 oz) tin tomatoes, chopped
½ tsp Worcester sauce
3 tbs thick plain yoghurt
3 tbs evaporated milk
salt and freshly ground black pepper, to taste
2 beef tomatoes, sliced
a little Parmesan cheese, grated

1. Flake the salmon into a shallow ovenproof dish.
2. Blend the tomato, Worcester sauce, yoghurt, evaporated milk and seasoning, and pour the mixture over the salmon.
3. Arrange the tomato slices over the top, followed by the Parmesan.
4. Bake at 350°F/180°C (Gas Mark 4) until the top is golden brown and bubbling (about 10 minutes).

Appetizers

Whitebait and Prawn Appetizer

150g (6 oz) celeriac, grated
1 heaped tbs plain low-fat yoghurt
tsp brown sugar
a little cider vinegar
225g (8 oz) whitebait
125g (4 oz) fresh, peeled prawns
olive or other vegetable oil, for frying

1. Make a celeriac salad by combining the grated celeriac
   with the yoghurt mixed with the sugar and enough of
   the cider vinegar to form a thinnish dressing. Chill the
   salad well.
2. Cook the whitebait and prawns in a little oil until the
   whitebait is crisp and the prawns have turned an even
   pink.
3. Serve them immediately with the chilled celeriac salad.

Baked Scallops

Scallops are not especially rich in EPA but they are very
popular as a starter, and a good way of getting friends and
family used to eating fish more often.

a little unsalted butter
4 large scallops
freshly ground black pepper, to taste
finely grated fresh white breadcrumbs

1. Lightly grease an ovenproof dish with a little of the butter
   and put the scallops in it, dotting them with small flakes
   of butter.
2. Season them with pepper and scatter just enough
   crumbs over them to coat them. Dot with a little more
   butter and bake in a 350°F/180°C (Gas Mark 4) oven for

about 20 minutes. The juices from the fish moisten the lower part of the crumbs, while the top layer becomes golden brown and crispy. Eat at once.

Soused Herrings

1 medium onion, finely chopped
2 large herring, filleted
about 900ml (1 pt) malt vinegar
450ml (½ pt) water
3 fresh or dried bay leaves
salt and freshly ground black pepper
1 tbs coriander seeds
1 tbs allspice berries
plenty of fresh parsley, chopped
brown bread, sliced and buttered, to serve

1. Preheat the oven to 300°F/150°C (Gas Mark 2).
2. Pack as much onion as you can inside the fish. Roll them up and fasten each one securely with a wooden toothpick.
3. Put them in an ovenproof dish and add the remaining ingredients, except the parsley and bread.
4. Bake the herrings in the preheated oven for 3 hours. Leave the fish to cool in the liquid, which will turn to jelly, then eat with the fresh brown bread and the chopped parsley.

Main meal

Fresh Grilled Sardines

This recipe is the essence of simplicity, using fresh, plain ingredients to their best advantage.

six medium tomatoes
salt and freshly ground black pepper
some fresh or dried basil to taste
450g (1 lb) fresh sardines
Tabasco sauce

1. Make the tomato salad by slicing the tomatoes thinly and sprinkling a very little salt over them to make the juices run, then pepper and a little basil to taste. Chill the salad for at least an hour.
2. Eat the salad with hot, grilled sardines, cooked with a couple of drops of Tabasco sauce on each fish, and some fresh, crusty granary bread or cooked rice.

Oatmealed Mackerel

Mackerel remains cheap and easy to find in fresh fish shops, so try this recipe.

2 mackerel
2 tbs medium oatmeal
olive oil, for frying
English mustard, to taste

1. Wipe the fish with damp kitchen paper, brush them with a little olive oil and coat them with the oatmeal.
2. Fry the fish gently in a little oil (some of the oatmeal is bound to come off, but is delicious scraped from the pan and served with the fish). Eat with a little of the English mustard.

Trout with Asparagus

You can use the 'asparagus pieces' for this recipe, which are cheaper. Tender new potatoes are the perfect accompaniment to the trout.

1 large or 2 medium field mushrooms, chopped
1×165g (6½ oz) tin of asparagus, drained
2 trout, filleted
olive oil, for frying
2 wedges of fresh lemon

1. Mix the mushrooms with the asparagus and put this inside the fish.
2. Fry the trout gently for about 10 minutes, turning them gently once. Squeeze the lemon juice from the wedges over the cooked fish.

Chapter 7

Exercising as a way of life

After diet comes exercise. This is rarely a popular topic and the thought of having to give up a largely sedentary way of life for one that includes regular, strenuous activity is enough to make many people wonder if it is all worth the bother. If *you* are wondering this, just take another look at the heart attack mortality figures in the first chapter, the growing numbers of women who are succumbing and the cardiovascular risk factors. These really should convince you that learning to exercise again is a small price to pay for good health.

I say 'again', for very few healthy young children lead a sedentary life and you can remember the time when you would literally 'run home from school' or 'up the road to the shops'. The fact that you had played football or netball at school that afternoon *and* had been for a cycle ride with your friends would in no way have deterred you.

Popular responses to these remarks include, 'Well, children have so much more energy' and 'I cannot expect to be as active as that at my age'. Children do, indeed, have a greater capacity for extremely vigorous activity – in short bursts – than older family members, who are more inclined in turn to have far greater stamina for prolonged exercise. 'But', you may be protesting '*which* adults? I cannot even pelt down the road after a bus like I did 10 years ago.' The answer that all healthy adults who have either never ceased to be physically energetic or who have deliberately set out to retrain their muscles and circulatory systems are leading a healthier way of life than the rest of us.

There is a certain amount of age-related decline in our available energy, but this is only a small part of the reason why many adults in Western society are thoroughly unfit. Stress, mental fatigue and often boredom during the day at work or in the home are generally relieved by food, alcohol, television or trips to the pub in the evening.

All these panaceas – food is certainly both necessity *and* panacea – are fine in their own way, but no substitute for a brisk, half-hour's walk or swim. There are few things so wearing as ennui and if your lifestyle is beginning to pall, then it is up to you to make it more exciting. How to do so will be explained in the next chapter. Taking regular exercise will increase your energy level, renew your enthusiasm for life and living, and pay dividends cosmetically. Believing the falsehood that 'I am getting on and am too unfit to exercise' will have the opposite effect and is the most dangerous attitude we can adopt.

It is really in trying to find the solution to an energy-sapping, lack-lustre lifestyle that the Five-point Plan finds its best application. All five elements – food, exercise, relaxation and recreation, ceasing to smoke and taking dietary supplements – are closely interconnected and interdependent. A healthy, wholefood diet, for instance – especially one with a raw content – increases vitality, improves one's looks and helps to combat stress. It also enables us to regain and maintain a normal body weight, and helps to guard against high blood pressure and a raised blood level of dangerous low density lipoproteins (LDL). Moreover, it provides energy for exercise.

Exercise of the aerobic variety has a whole range of beneficial effects. It tones up the muscles, especially that of the heart, keeps joints, tendons and ligaments flexible and supple, burns up excess calories and helps maintain a healthy appetite. It combats and offers protection against arthritis. Most important in the present context, it helps to keep blood pressure and the LDL blood level low. The cardiovascular system as a whole becomes healthier and less 'accident prone' and sleep and relaxation are more thorough and restful.

Rest and relaxation are, without doubt, more beneficial when our bodily systems are in good working order. Deep, tranquil sleep is achieved by following a proper relaxation technique, and this can be learned either in classes or at home. You are far more likely to wake up refreshed and ready to tackle another day when you have learned, quite literally, how to 'recreate' yourself and how to switch off. Relaxation methods, in turn, are aided by a healthy diet, supplements, regular exercise of the right kind and ceasing to rely on nicotine to 'steady your nerves'.

Supplements supply those nutrients we need in the correct proportions. They are essential for optimum health and many have long-lasting effects in the body which scientists believe help to keep us young and active. Some, such as pure fish oil containing EPA, offer protection from life-threatening conditions.

The benefits of giving up smoking of tobacco in any form are clear to many people, including the majority of smokers. We will see in a later chapter how to come face to face with your dependence on tobacco and how to *want*, really and truly, to be free from it for good. Determination and will-power are more than half the secret of success.

Research studies

There is ample proof that regular exercise reduces the risk of having a heart attack. A very interesting early study, carried out by the Medical Research Council, compared the number of heart attacks suffered by workers with sedentary jobs with those affecting postmen on delivery rounds. The physically active workers had less than half the number of heart attacks of their less active comrades.

Many other epidemiological studies conducted since this early famous one have confirmed these findings, showing that the heart and the cardiovascular system as a whole clearly benefit from regular exercise. People who are health conscious and eager to decrease their own families' health risks are understandably far keener to change their lifestyle – which is always a momentous undertaking – provided they can see the sense of doing so. Consistent epidemiological study results are convincing and indicative in a broad sense of what will and will not keep us healthy. More to the point, perhaps, at a personal level, is the explanation of just how and why these benefits accrue.

Heartfelt benefits

1. Stronger, healthier heart

A feature in a Sunday newspaper magazine described the ways in which a number of thalidomide victims – now adults – cope with their daily lives. Most of them coped marvellously and one felt the greatest admiration for the ingenious ways in which they managed to overcome their handicaps. One young woman was especially memorable. She worked as a groom, having in her charge a stable of show jumpers and a coloured photograph showed her, not only jumping one of the horses, which she managed to control by means of reins connected with her feet, but also to tack her horses up. Lacking arms, she made most use of her legs, feet and flipper hands. Her large toe on one foot, it was commented, had developed enormously in size and strength and, in many ways, played the part of an extra hand.

The reason for this augmented development was the extra burden the toe had been encouraged to bear over and above what is normally expected of a large toe. The more you use a particular muscle or group of muscles, the more their substance and strength will grow to achieve what is being expected of them. A familiar example of this 'growth in proportion to use' is the enormous muscular development apparent in weightlifters and athletes. 'Bodybuilding' would have no visible effects if it did not increase the muscles of the torso, arms and legs to such extreme extents.

The heart – which, after all, is simply a highly ingenious muscle – responds in the same way. Two young men aged 25, for instance, one of whom is a cross-country runner and the other of whom is a 'sit-in-the-chair-in-front-of-the-telly' man will have different-sized hearts relative to the different demands made upon them by their owners. The runner's heart will be bigger and stronger and able to pump far more blood per beat in what is called its 'stroke volume' than that of the armchair TV enthusiast.

As both men will have the same volume of blood, fewer beats per minute are required by the fit man's heart to pump it round the body. This is why his pulse rate may well be in the region of 55 to 65 beats per minute, while that of his friend is more likely to lie between 75 and 85 beats per minute. The effect of this is fewer heartbeats per 24 hours, which in turn means more resting time. This improves the arterial blood supply to the heart, since blood flows through the coronary arteries and out into the substance of the heart, only during the rest phase between contractions.

In addition, frequent demands upon the heart increase the internal capacity of these arteries. They get used to transporting the larger volumes of blood needed when exercise is being taken and they also expand readily in response to the chemical stimulants released by the muscle fibres of the heart when exercise is being taken. Clots are less likely to form, too, when blood spends relatively little time trickling through the arteries concerned and more in pouring through in a greatly increased volume.

2. Lower blood fat levels

Blood fat levels, especially those of the low density atheroma-forming variety, increase in response to stress. A study of final year medical students with an average age of 23 years, showed that levels of dangerous LDL rose in response to stress, both before exams and before representing their college in an inter-university quiz. Interestingly, the levels were higher among the women than among the men immediately before a viva (oral) exam and higher among the men before a written paper. There was no difference between the elevated blood fat levels of either sex immediately prior to the verbal quiz contest.

Acute anxiety, as well as the more prolonged, chronic type that arises in connection with mortgages and marital affairs rather than exams and tests, elevates LDL blood levels in this way by the effect of adrenaline and noradrenaline. These two hormones are secreted by the adrenal glands when a challenging situation is faced and, among other effects, mobilize fat in the form of globules from the body's excess stores. This may be one of the reasons why physical thinness is associated with chronic worry.

The surplus fat circulates in the bloodstream, ready to supply extra energy where and when needed, in order that appropriate physical action can be taken in view of the threat being posed. The problem is few anxiety-making situations in our present society warrant physical action, either aggressive or defensive. Getting behind with mortgage repayments can only be solved by increasing one's income or channelling funds directed elsewhere towards the Building Society's accounts department. For this reason, the excessive amounts of fat – at the ready to help cope with the dilemma – are not actually needed. They are, however, available in the blood for that most unwanted of functions – the deposition in the walls of arteries to build further atheromatous plaque.

Frequent, brisk exercise boosts the blood levels of the protective, safe, high density lipoproteins (HDLs). Men and women who take such exercise have a very greatly reduced risk of suffering from ischaemic disease. Getting fit by gradually re-introducing regular physical activity into your life also lowers the level of the low density type and, if maintained, slowly erodes the fibrous atheromatous plaques, thereby unclogging arteries that may have been furred up for years.

3. A decreased tendency to form blood clots

Vigorous exercise, such as playing singles tennis or swimming as fast as you can, even if carried out for only five to ten minutes, increases the 'fibrinolytic' chemical action of the blood. The other context in which we have met the process of fibrinolysis is when looking at the action of prostaglandins. Some prostaglandins, like thromboxane, enhance the clotting mechanism and others, like prostacycline, counteract this effect, (in other words their reaction is thrombolytic).

The thrombolytic activity that results from exercise lasts for 60 to 70 minutes after the exercise has ceased. Unlike drugs designed to prevent thrombosis, exercise, when properly carried out, has only beneficial effects.

4. Lowers blood pressure

Like a raised blood fat level, blood pressure can become elevated in response to persistent stress, combined with a sedentary lifestyle, particularly when found in conjunction with obesity, smoking and a high-fat/salt/sugar, low-fibre diet. Exercise lowers tension and stress and permits action to be taken that at least *represents* and gives release to the violent 'fight or flight' activity for which our adrenal glands prepare us. Pounding round the block in a way that challenges heart and arteries or playing badminton, squash or hockey, help the 'tightly coiled spring within' to uncoil and the blood pressure to fall.

We saw in an earlier discussion, that essential hypertension is thought to start with spasm of the small arteries of the body in response to stress and/or other factors. Raised blood pressure, present over a period of time, is then believed to damage the lining of these small vessels, which in turn become permanently narrowed within – thereby increasing the blood pressure.

As well as enabling you to cope with emotional tension in a realistic and healthy way, exercise of the right type, performed regularly, reduces your body weight to normal – normal being that which is metabolically optimal for you as an individual. The majority of overweight people have higher blood pressure than their slim peers, because the heart has a heavier work load. Often simply losing weight is all that is required for the correction of their hypertension.

Ought you to exercise?

Hopefully, I have said enough in this chapter to convince you that exercise is vital if you want to steer clear of heart and arterial disease. If you or a family member already suffers from angina or has experienced a heart attack, you may feel very differently about it. The medical facts show, however, that the only way back to health is by way of exercise – the sort of exercise that makes tangible demands upon your heart and lungs.

Exercise therapy in the management of anginal pain has been examined in a number of clinical studies. In one of these, ten patients took part, with angina severity ranging from mild to moderately severe. After one year of carefully controlled and gradually developing exercises, seven patients were entirely free of angina and the other three had improved considerably, both in frequency of attacks and in their severity.

The essential thing to bear in mind, whether you already

suffer from some form of arterial or ischaemic heart disease or are merely unfit, is *do not go at it hammer and tongs*. Here are some tips for easing yourself pleasurably into your new routine.

● Ask your doctor for a checkup, telling him or her why you need one. Your best course of action is to have a word with the receptionist and suggest that you be given a double appointment. Many doctors feel a bit flummoxed on being asked for a checkup during the usual consultation time of 5 to 10 minutes, as the word – being so non-specific – conjures up time-consuming examinations of the central nervous system and entire body musculature. Also, what any particular patient means by a checkup, usually depends entirely upon which 'medical book for the layman' he or she has most recently read.

The essentials for your requirements are: a pulse check, a thorough, even if brief, listen to your heart and lungs, a blood pressure check, a weight check if you even suspect you may be overweight and an ECG if you have had any form of heart disease, diabetes or hypertension. The ECG should include a stress test, that is, an ECG tracing performed after you have been exerting yourself physically. This is normally performed at a special centre or clinic to which your GP can send you.

Ask for your blood fat levels to be checked as well. It will be interesting – and rewarding – to watch the levels of the dangerous low density variety fall as you succeed in making regular exercise a part of your lifestyle. Ask for the level to be checked every three to six months, together with your weight and blood pressure.

● As Donald Norfolk says succinctly in his admirable book, *Fit For Life* (Hamlyn Paperbacks, 1981), 'Remember that the aim of cardiovascular conditioning programmes is to train, not to strain.' I enthusiastically endorse this advice as, quite apart from the physical damage that may result from taking over-violent exercise after years of a sedentary lifestyle, your enthusiasm is likely to be badly dampened by the inevitable failure of your body to respond to your overtaxing demands. The road ahead to fitness can then look too long, thorny and desolate and the familiar armchair even more seductive than usual. Many over-zestful would-be keep fitters fizzle out in this way.

Be sure to limber up before doing any exercise and do not underestimate the importance of a cooling down session at the end. This means stopping hectic exercise *gradually*, tailing it off over a period of minutes and moving about gently, as you pack your gear, shower, change and do your hair. Do not simply stop with no warning to your system. Your circulation needs time to readjust from your requirements while exercising to your requirements once you have ceased to exercise. Walk briskly before you even attempt to jog and be content with swimming a couple of lengths at first, even though your aim is ultimately to swim 20.

● Finally, make sure that you enjoy whatever type of exercise you mean to take up. If you intend to learn something new, find out about it first, and have a few trial runs before taking it up seriously. Just as important, fit your exercise into a part of the day when other demands are least likely to be made on you. It is enough to have to keep your eye on your watch, making sure that you work out for whatever interval you have chosen. You do not want to feel anxious, at the same time, that you may be missing an important telephone call or that the baby may be crying.

Aerobic exercise

Aerobic exercise is the type of exercise you have to take in order to get all the benefits so far mentioned. 'Aerobic' in this context simply means that the exercise taken increases

Fish Oil

the need of the bodily organs for oxygen and glucose fuel. This is the only way to improve the functional ability of the heart, blood vessels and lungs. You can tell when you are exercising aerobically, because your heart beat will increase and you will breathe more rapidly in an attempt to keep up supplies to cope with your increased oxygen requirement.

Age	Max. heart rate	Exercise rate if fit beats per minute	Exercise rate if unfit beats per minute
16	204	164	123
18	202	162	122
20	200	160	120
22	198	158	119
24	196	157	118
26	194	155	116
28	192	154	115
30	190	152	114
32	188	151	113
34	186	149	112
36	184	148	110
38	182	146	109
40	180	144	108
45	175	140	105
50	170	136	102
55	165	132	99
60	160	128	96
65	155	124	93

Table 1   Exercising pulse rates by age and fitness

Aerobic exercise also increases your 'metabolic rate', that is, the rate at which you burn fuel and, provided you keep up your activity for 30 minutes or longer, you will gain the added bonus of an increased metabolic rate persisting for some time after you cease to exercise. In other words, you burn up extra calories while you exercise and this increased rate of fuel (that is, excess fat) consumption continues afterwards while you rest. (If you are not at all overweight, you have very little excess fat to lose. To avoid losing any of your lean body mass (muscular tissue), increase the proportion of complex carbohydrates in your diet, as outlined in the previous chapter.)

Pulse rate

Once you have decided to swim, jog, horse-ride, skip or otherwise get yourself fit, keep a careful eye upon your pulse rate. This is a useful, and vital, means of both monitoring your progress and making certain that you are demanding enough of your body to make your effort worthwhile, without demanding too much and straining your heart. The maximum heart rate you should reach is calculated by subtracting your age from 220. To benefit from aerobic exercise, you should allow your pulse to reach 60 per cent of this figure if you are unfit and 80 per cent if you are fit. Table 1 shows the correct training rates according to age and fitness. Refer to the higher of two ages if you are between two of them.

Beats per minute	
Under 60 — very fit	80–90 — below average
60–70 — fit	Over 90 — unfit
70–80 — average	

Table 2   Resting pulse rate fitness guide

Your pulse at rest indicates your present state of fitness and this is best measured first thing in the morning before eating or drinking (see Table 2). Remember that fear, stress, alcohol, fever, tea, coffee and certain drugs can increase your resting pulse rate artificially. Check your pulse, too, 5 minutes after you stop exercising: it ought not to exceed 120 beats a minute – if it does, you have exercised too hard. Take it more slowly next time.

Fish Oil

12 *minutes*	15 *minutes*	20 *minutes*
Running on the spot	Jogging	Brisk walking
Skipping	Distance running	Cycling
Trampolining	Rowing	Skating
Competitive swimming	Dancing	Swimming

Table 3   Minimum workout times

It is necessary to exercise for a certain number of minutes to obtain full 'aerobic' benefits. The chart given in Table 3 indicates the minimum workout times. Once you are fitter, exercise for at least 20 minutes, preferably 30 to 40, three or four times weekly.

Chapter 8

Giving up smoking

It has already been shown that we run an increased risk of having a heart attack if we smoke. The trial mentioned in Chapter 1 involved male subjects, but I also pointed out the increased risk run by women of suffering from ischaemic heart disease once they have reached menopause. Over the past 15 years, the incidence of heart attacks among women has increased – the especially dangerous combinations of risk factors being the contraceptive Pill + cigarettes or the post-menopausal period + cigarettes. Either of these combined with a sedentary lifestyle, obesity and a high-fat diet, further multiply the chances of dying from a coronary thrombosis.

There are fewer women smokers in the UK than there used to be, mainly because many older women have given up the habit, although more teenage girls than ever are taking to it. Ironically, smoking brings about an earlier menopause in many women, so the protection against heart disease afforded by a high level of natural oestrogen in the blood is lost sooner than it might otherwise be. In addition, unborn babies can be affected by their mothers smoking during pregnancy. On average, their weight is lower and they seem to get off to a poorer start in life, being extra prone to chest infections.

Lethal chemicals

Perhaps you have seen either the play or the film of Shakespeare's Egyptian Queen. Lovely and beguiling, Cleopatra appeared goddess-like to Mark Antony who, forsaking comrades and honour to cleave only to her, ended by falling on his sword – having learned too late the evil of which she was capable. None – not even the mightiest and most notable general – was spared the injury that could ensue from amorous contact with her. So also nicotine, sometimes referred to as 'the Goddess', offers those who pursue her great pleasure, calm nerves and a 'prop' when they feel in need – all the while silently wreaking deadly harm.

Nicotine is a highly dangerous alkaloid poison. It is one of more than 2,000 chemicals present in tobacco smoke and, like many of the others, is transported around the body in the bloodstream which it enters while within the lungs. While coal tar deposits are responsible for cancer of the lungs and sometimes of the tongue and throat, nicotine affects the nerve endings of sympathetic and para-sympathetic nerves (the autonomic nervous system) which control the action of the heart, the behaviour of the blood vessels, the digestive functions and all the other 'automatic' activities within the body over which we have no direct control.

When you first take up the habit of smoking tobacco, it is the parasympathetic nerves that seem to be affected predominantly and the results may include intense nausea and vomiting, pallor and shakiness. Having got used to the drug, however, the sympathetic effects take over, and you experience pleasure and a feeling of calmness, although the harmful effects within this feeling include a fast pulse, raised blood pressure and poor appetite and digestion. Most dangerous of all, nicotine constricts blood vessels, *especially the coronary arteries,* and also increases the heart muscles' oxygen requirement. It is surely not necessary to paint a graphic picture of the effects of nicotine upon a heart whose coronary arteries are already partially clogged by atheromatous plaque, especially when other factors such as excitement or increased physical activity, are at the same time increasing the heart's need for oxygen.

The second 'horror story' ingredient of tobacco smoke is carbon monoxide – the very gas with which many successful suicides are committed, being a major component of petrol exhaust fumes. Carbon monoxide in high concentration kills outright by combining with the coloured pigment in the blood (haemoglobin) instead of oxygen. In the concentration in which it is present in tobacco smoke, carbon monoxide succeeds in combining to a significant degree with haemoglobin. In so doing, it also, like nicotine, increases the myocardium's need for oxygen.

In fact, when only 5 per cent of the haemoglobin has combined with carbon monoxide in place of oxygen, the coronary arteries need to transport 20 per cent more oxygen to the myocardial heart muscle to cater for its increased need. Diseased coronary arteries are rarely capable of doing this. Moreover, smoking increases the rate at which atheromatous plaque formation occurs, especially within the coronary arteries and encourages blood platelets to clump thus increasing the risk of thrombosis. The intimate connection between angina, heart attacks and smoking should now be clear! Imagine the cries of outrage that would result if a new type of addictive confectionery with the same effects as nicotine and carbon monoxide were introduced into the country.

How to stop smoking

There are a vast number of different ways in which you can stop smoking – for good. Like slimming diets, the method chosen and used by any particular person must be tailored to his or her needs, personality and lifestyle. Whereas gritting one's teeth and crash dieting may suit strong-willed people with quite a bit of weight to lose, so giving up cigarettes 'cold turkey' will suit some smokers and prove impossible to others.

Whatever method you choose, three factors are necessary for your success. These are *willpower, confidence and courage*. If any of these is lacking then you will be half-stopping, starting, totally stopping and restarting again after a week, for months or years, until you finally give up trying to stop altogether. Plenty of people join this bandwagon and, generally, at least with respect to their smoking habits, their self-regard and self-confidence is round about the level of their boots. The problem becomes like that of people who fail their driving test time and time again. Ultimately failure seems inevitable to them.

Willpower

Firstly, you must really *want* to stop smoking. This may seem too obvious for words, but many people purport to give up tobacco smoking because their friends are doing so, because they are short of cash for a while, because their husband or wife nags them into it or because they are made to feel a social outcast in restaurants, in places of indoor entertainment and on public transport.

Nicotine is strongly addictive and to say that a *fervent* desire to escape its death-embrace is essential, is not to state the case too strongly. Only if you, of yourself, are convinced of the dangers involved of getting cancer or ischaemic heart disease and of your moral duty not to force others into 'passive smoking' will you stand a good chance of success.

Confidence

People *do* give up cigarettes, cigars and pipe smoking for good – even people who have smoked 40 cigarettes or more all their adult lives. There is no reason on earth why you should not do so and of this truth you must convince yourself. My own personal recommendation is to make sure you do not allow this precious self-confidence to become eroded. Try once without professional help. Perhaps try a second time without professional help, if there was a very good reason that no longer applies, why you failed (sudden emotional upset, extra stress at work, for example). After that, seek out and pay for assistance in attaining your objective.

Courage

You will need this in plenty and not only because you will be fighting an addictive drug. You have to be prepared for family or friends to laugh at you, to be sceptical about your chances of success (especially if you have failed in the past) and deliberately to tempt you to start smoking again. Your response to this prediction may be, 'With friends like that, who needs enemies?' – and you may be luckier than most. Unfortunately it is part of human nature to joke at the expense of others, especially when there is an underlying feeling of guilt, self-doubt and envy on their part.

Have you ever tried dieting, only to have your fattest friend insist you are 'all right as you are' and show her contempt for slimming by pressing you to a jam and cream doughnut? Expect, therefore, for cigarette packets to be whipped out and offered to you whenever you appear, for people to ask you derisively, 'How many days is it now?' and for remarks to be made such as 'Smoking never harmed my old Dad – he lived to be 106 and smoked 30 cigarettes a day from the age of 12'. It should be pointed out that such cases are extremely rare.

Self-help method

Many experts say that you should avoid giving up smoking at a time of extra stress. Marital breakup, illness in the family, problems at work, even going on holiday (especially if you are frightened of flying) are all likely to increase your desire to smoke. It *is* harder under such circumstances, which is why I mentioned that failing then should not ruin your self-confidence, but it is wisest not to tax your system with potently toxic chemicals when it is already bearing the brunt of extra stress factors. Although you may have to fight harder to quit smoking when life is problematical, your sense of personal achievement when you have succeeded, added to your improved health and extra money in your pocket, can be expected to more than compensate.

Here are some aids to giving up smoking alone. Make a list of all the advantages you will gain – all the benefits to health, self-confidence and financial state that you can think of. Keep this somewhere handy and read it through daily. Tell whomever you live with that you intend to quit, if you can rely on their help. Alternatively, keep your intention a secret and, if asked, reply vaguely that 'you do not really fancy a cigarette just now – you may have a cold coming on'. This is not a lie, anyone *may* have a cold coming on. Incidentally, an infection of the upper respiratory tract provides an excellent opportunity to give up smoking. A sore throat and/or head cold generally makes cigarettes taste vile, so take full advantage of such an occasion should it arise.

Then, either simply decide at the end of your present packet not to buy any more or cut down over a period of time that seems appropriate to you – say, over a week if you smoke 10 cigarettes daily, over a fortnight if you smoke 20 a day or over three weeks if you smoke more than this. Try not to extend your 'quitting period' beyond 21 days, though, as the temptation then arises simply to cut *down* instead of cutting *out*.

With respect to craving cigarettes when you are withdrawing from nicotine, try taking extra exercise as described in the last chapter. I am not writing this as one who has never smoked, but as one who knows the difficulties very well, having experienced them. The point about exercise is that doing something actively tiring takes your mind off the smoking urge and often bolsters your self-esteem enough for the craving not to return for several hours.

In addition, if you have been breathless recently, your breathing will improve at least in part when you stop smoking. You will find that after only a few days taking exercise becomes a more welcome thought and you are feeling better for it. This is a very good feeling indeed. If your breathing does not improve as you lose weight and stop smoking, then visit your doctor again for a further check. Try, also, some of the relaxation suggestions which you will find in the next chapter. These are a very efficient way of banishing the 'reaching-screaming-pitch' feeling.

Lastly, if you do need a chemical prop, take a very small amount of supplementary nicotine to tide you over the worst of the withdrawal craving. Chemists sell a variety, one brand name being *Stoppers*. Alternatively, get your doctor to prescribe *Nicorette* chewing gum, for which you will have to pay the retail price and chew it strictly according to the instructions. Various herbal remedies exist and a good idea is to ask your chemist or health food shop retailer about them. Potters' *Anti-Smoking Tablets* contain 32.5mg of the herb lobelia, well-known in herbal lore to help combat the smoking habit. These have to be taken in a dose of one or two every two hours and sucked for 30 minutes, after which time you swallow them whole.

Leslie and Susannah Kenton, in *Raw Energy* (Century, 1985), mention that chewing sunflower seeds is a help when giving up smoking. These are very nutritious as they contain vitamins, minerals, EFAs and protein, and have a pleasant flavour. Alternatively, or in addition to these ideas, you can try the special cigarette filters (which normally come in a box of four). You use one a week for four weeks, which is a bit long, but they are useful in that they successively filter off more and more of the cigarette smoke's ingredients, including the nicotine, so that you accustom yourself gradually to doing without it.

Hypnotic suggestion

Hypnosis – known properly as hypnotherapy – can be used very effectively to help patients relinquish unwanted habits. Hypnotherapy is not usually available on the National Health, but GPs are often happy to refer suitable patients to practitioners known personally to them and others practise the art themselves.

If your GP cannot help you, look in the Yellow Pages under 'Hypnotherapists', 'Therapy' or 'Psychotherapists'. Look for letters after the therapist's name and if you do not know what they stand for, do not be scared to ask. LNCP, for instance, stands for Licentiate of the National Council of Psychotherapists and Hypnotherapists. (You can locate the practitioner in your area, trained by that school, by contacting the Chairman, W. Broom Esq, 46 Oxhey Road, Oxhey, Watford WD1 4QQ (Tel: 0923-227772).

There is insufficient space here to describe how hypnosis works in terms that would do it justice. Suffice it to say that the modern practice of hypnotherapy has travelled light years from the time when the only hypnosis known to most people was that of the stage hypnotist. The purpose of hypnotic trance is neither to dominate your personality, nor to learn your innermost secrets. You cannot be ordered to do that which is morally reprehensible to you – brainwashing and the art of hypnotherapy are as far apart as the wanton destruction of human beings by bomb attacks and the patient, skilful mending of their maimed bodies by experienced surgeons.

Having assured you upon the points most people are worried about, here is some practical information you may find useful. Wanting to give up smoking is one of the most common problems that hypnotherapists deal with and most have adopted specific treatment regimes which, in their experience, are most effective. One method, for instance, involves a single session in which the therapist will implant an idea called a 'post-hypnotic suggestion' in your subconscious mind. The likely form for such a suggestion is that, from then onwards, cigarettes would taste and smell of whatever particular substance you have mentioned earlier as disgusts you.

The range of possibilities is enormous, since one man's or woman's meat really is another's poison. Some patients find the smell and look of ripe, blue cheese completely repulsive, while others are revolted by urine, sewage, rotting meat or silage. These suggestions may sound pretty strong, but the aim of this trance suggestion is to cause aversion to the cigarettes to which you are addicted. A deeply rooted habit can require powerful tools to remove it.

A second technique frequently used is the 'Q day method' in which 'Q' or 'Quitting day' is the last of four weekly appointments. Post-hypnotic suggestions are implanted at each preceding session, enabling you to wean yourself gradually off cigarettes by smoking fewer and fewer each week until you finally stop altogether. The cost of a session is usually in the region of £15–£30, a small price to pay for the benefits to your health and well-being.

Chapter 9

Combating the harmful effects of stress

Stress is renowned for making most health problems worse. There is no doubt that it is a serious risk factor in heart disease, as was shown in the first chapter in the discussion both of stress itself and of personality types. Just to restate the seriousness of its effects, chronic (that is, persistent) stress keeps the cells throughout our bodies permanently geared for the 'flight or fight' response, even though it is very rare for either reaction to solve the problem.

We remain in this supercharged, 'ready to fly off the handle' state because our adrenal glands are being stimulated by the stress factors we encounter to secrete large amounts of the two hormones adrenaline and noradrenaline. These increase our pulse rate, constrict many of our smaller arteries, thereby increasing our blood pressure, elevate our blood fat level, partially block the formation of helpful prostaglandins of the E1 series, derived from the dietary EFA linoleic acid and elevate our output of prostaglandins of the E2 series which collectively *increase* fibrous atheromatous plaque and blood clot formation.

Types of stress

With all these adverse reactions to stress, it seems remarkable at first that any of us ever survive our first 20 to 30 years of life! One might wonder that the mortality rate from heart and arterial disease is not double its present level and be puzzled by the fact that a high blood cholesterol reading rather than stress remains at the top of the list of cardiovascular disease risk factors.

However, many things capable of inflicting serious harm in certain situations are of benefit when we encounter them in other circumstances. This is one of the principles underlying the science and art of homoeopathic medicine. Arsenic, for instance, notoriously lethal when taken in any quantity, is useful in the treatment (among other complaints) of heart disease and circulatory problems when administered in minute quantities.

Stress works in the same way. Although one of the dictionary definitions of stress is: 'A mentally or emotionally disruptive or disquieting influence', it depends very much upon both the quality and the quantity of the stress you encounter. Not all stress is injurious and small amounts of the right type of stress are, in fact, essential to our development and continuing vitality. 'Good' forms of stress include challenges in which we voluntarily engage, such as those encountered at work, in our studies and in sport and pastimes. These occur at all levels and within the lifestyle structures of every one of us.

At one end of the 'useful' stress spectrum we may place an advertising executive applying for the post of Accounts Director. If fit and capable, then he or she will probably secretly enjoy providing a perfectly presented CV, writing a persuasive letter of application, buying new clothes for the interview and competing with other contenders on the appointed day. At the other end of the spectrum, we can place a small child trying, failing, and finally learning, to tie a bow, pull on his socks or do up his coat buttons for the first time ever.

Further examples of stress chosen at random across the human spectrum show its infinite variety and application. A little old lady, collecting and arranging some wild flowers for a Women's Institute competition, a 40-year-old woman, who hasn't ridden a horse since she was 15, taking up the sport once more and a member of the Shadow Cabinet, working to further both his Party's aims, as well as his own objective, which is to accede to the Premiership at the next election. All these are instances of stress – good, healthy, life-enhancing stress at a purely personal level.

Good stress makes you feel like a million dollars. It puts a spring into your step and zest into your appetite – both for food and for love. It brings colour to your cheeks and it makes your eyes sparkle. You feel 20, 30, 50 or 80 years *young*, not old, and life is worth living. How, then, can some stress be a killer?

Notice that I define useful stresses as the ones we take upon ourselves voluntarily. In fact, even some of those we do not seek, such as a suddenly increased work load at the office, four guests arriving for dinner when one's partner has forgotten to mention inviting them and an unexpected request one 'cannot refuse' to make a public speech, can all improve our sense of well-being by increasing our sense of self-worth – provided we do not panic and make a mess of things. It is whether or not we learn to *handle* stress constructively that determines whether it is to have a health-promoting effect upon us or bring us tangibly closer to suffering a heart attack.

Harmful stress

Some of us are able to cope with prolonged periods of stress without coming to any harm. Others go weak at the knees after relatively brief periods of stressful experience. To further complicate elucidation of the whole stress picture are the facts that *certain* forms of physical and emotional trauma, especially when they strike in combined force, take a severe toll of even the most relaxed people and certain individuals make matters worse for themselves by repressing their natural reactions to traumatic life events.

Among the highest rated stress factors are death of one's partner, bereavement of any other family member or a close friend, loss of employment, divorce or separation from one's partner, financial problems, moving house, changing jobs – even Christmas is fairly high on the official stress list. This may come as a surprise at first, but when you come to think about it, the Christmas 'break' often runs close to being precisely that! Far from offering most people in our society a chance to experience 'peace on earth and good will to all men', it manages to pack more stress factors into the 48 hours of Christmas Day and Boxing Day, than many of us encounter for weeks on end!

I think the stress factor list ought to re-state 'Christmas' as 'the Christmas period'. Many people become so anxious and exhausted during the fortnight of frenetic activity prior to 'the great day', that they are incapable of coping with the sudden demands of over-excited children, fractious in-laws and elaborate food preparation that the 'holiday period' entails. It is small wonder that the number of patients admitted to coronary care units each year between Christmas Eve and New Year is as high as it is.

Types of stress factors that inevitably affect people in a serious fashion are sudden illness or accidents befalling either themselves or a family member, the prolonged care of a sick or disabled relative, child or partner, serious financial loss and bereavement. When, in some unfortunate individuals, one or several of these coincide with, perhaps, sudden redundancy or dismissal from work, buying and selling a house, a family quarrel and severe marital strain, it brings home to helpless onlookers just how lacerating 'the slings and arrows of outrageous fortune' can be.

Of those admirable people who seem to carry on regardless, however much emotional and physical buffeting they receive, some are past masters at coping with crises and usually manage to emerge from periods of appalling strain, wiser, stronger and more philosophical than they had been previously. In other words, they turn severe stress to their advantage. Others repress the pain, anger and fear they feel under an outer mask of resilient capability, while within they are giving free rein to high-level stress to wreak as much havoc as it is capable of – which is a lot.

In reality, they are *increasing* their already considerable problems by adding an inner conflict to their sum total of stress. This conflict stems from a personality and unbringing that insist upon the retention of a 'stiff upper lip' at all costs, regardless of how heavy the latter may be. Instead of finding a healthy outlet for their grief and fury, they quietly develop high blood pressure, extensive atherosclerosis, angina and often thrombosis and become highly likely candidates for either a heart attack or a stroke.

In addition to these cardiovascular problems, one should also remember the other stress-related disorders to which they become prey. These include peptic ulceration, spastic colon, colitis and diverticulitis, chronic digestive problems, certain forms of cancer, a lowered pain threshold, tension headaches and migraine attacks, muscular aches and pains, sexual problems, a decreased resistance to infectious illnesses, depression and other psychiatric problems. Symptoms and signs of losing the stress battle include insomnia, chronic fatigue, appetite abnormalities (either loss of interest in food or the inability to leave it alone), reduced interest in both job, family and social life, poor concentration and diminished output and feelings of intense irritability that become difficult to control.

The role of personality

People who react poorly to stress use various means, either consciously or unconsciously, to lessen the strain upon themselves. The 'poor copers' include two types of people. First, those who go to pieces as soon as their burden grows too heavy to bear. This is 'coping' in a way, because in most causes a violent reaction to stress results in emergency treatment often including hospitalization, with the consequent removal, at least for the present, of the overwhelming problem. Second, there are those who increase their adverse reactions to stress by refusing to provide a healthy outlet for them.

Besides the 'A' and 'B' personality factors involved, there is also the question of nationality. English people are especially good at remaining superficially phlegmatic and unruffled, while harbouring strong emotions within. There is a lot to be said, health-wise, for the more volatile Mediterranean temperament, that reacts violently whenever upset, and rarely maintains a calm exterior when hurt, insulted or shocked.

As was mentioned in the discussion of fish-eating habits, Mediterranean people have a considerably lower incidence of cardiovascular disease than we do in the UK. Perhaps – in addition to oily fish consumption – their passionate natures play an important role in keeping their hearts and arteries free of disease. The British have been called 'the salt of the earth' and, to extend the condiment analogy, one could say that the Southern French, Italians, Spanish and Portuguese temperaments have more in common with chilli peppers.

Salt plays a vital role in the healthy human organism. However, too much of it is actually a risk factor in developing high blood pressure, whereas chilli pepper is renowned for its ability both to stimulate the digestion and to induce a mood of euphoria! As is usually the case in nature, harmony is attained by achieving a perfect balance and the best combination is most probably small but equal pinches of the two of them within the human personality!

Anti-stress tactics to avoid

Many people under stress, whatever category they fall into, increase their overall health problems by turning to tobacco, drinking more alcohol, tea or coffee, overeating and taking even less exercise than usual. Turning to such activities for comfort is a very understandable human response and one in which we all indulge from time to time. Unfortunately, these 'outlets' are bad for our health when taken individually, while, if indulged in collectively, they can prove fatal.

- **Cigarettes** There is no need to reiterate the dangers to the heart and arteries, of smoking tobacco as these have already been dealt with in detail. (See Chapter 8.)
- **Alcohol**, however, is a two-edged sword. It can be a trusty friend when taken socially in small amounts. It 'breaks the ice' at parties and social gatherings, helps you to relax and reduces the impact – temporarily – of an intolerably unfriendly world. Between 1 and 2 units daily have been shown actually to afford some protection against heart attacks, where a unit is a single measure of spirits, liqueur, fortified wine or sherry, or half a pint of beer or lager, or a 5-fluid ounce glass of table wine. The recommended maximum intake for a man is 21 units per week and 14 for a woman.

  Taken in larger quantities as an emotional 'prop' or specifically to relieve chronic stress, though, alcohol is a deadly enemy. Its effects bring to mind the time-honoured warning, 'Beware of the Greeks as they come, bearing gifts.' Alcohol *lures* one into believing it is a friendly, reliable disposer of worry and care. Meanwhile, as you grow more and more eager for your evening glass or four of your favourite tipple, it is building up your dependence upon it, adversely affecting your liver and brain cells, putting up your weekly financial outgoings, probably creating or increasing domestic disharmony and adding hundreds of worthless calories to your daily energy intake.

  An increase in weight not only overtaxes your heart, puts up your blood pressure and poses other health problems, it can devastate your sense of self-worth and enormously increases your stress and misery. Consequently, you add even more alcohol to your daily intake, in a vain attempt to overcome the added stress.

● **Food** Whereas some of us turn to the bottle to relieve emotional misery, others turn to *food*. Generally, in the case of inveterate pickers and snackers, *any* food will serve the purpose. Whatever one thinks of Freudian theory, most people would admit that much oral pleasure – satisfying at a deeply emotional level – can be derived from contact between the lips and mouth and something pleasant to suck or chew.

Whether or not this awakens early memories of the breast or bottle in years gone by, food – especially sweet, gooey, sticky junk snacks – can provide a tremendous amount of satisfaction and reassuring comfort. Ironically, just one of the points of comfort about eating is that at least food is always there (at least in our society) and can be relied upon in times of need, however one's friends, lover or family might treat one.

The bathroom scales and one's present wardrobe of clothes are quick to bear witness to the destructiveness of this behaviour – not to mention our rapidly diminishing fitness as we struggle, panting, up stairs that in the past we have run up without a second thought. When this state of affairs threatens to arise, the time to seek professional help is *immediately*. This is equally true if alcohol has started to pose even a hint of a problem.

(I feel bound to add the 'rider' that I do, very occasionally, indulge in a junk snack and am no supporter of the 'alcohol-is-a-sin' Band of Hope lobby. I take the greatest delight in a triple Cinzano Bianco on crushed ice whenever I have something exciting to celebrate. So I am not pontificating from some privileged position, far removed from the frailties of human flesh. I have simply, as a doctor, seen enough of the human misery that alcoholism, eating disorders *and* heart disease can cause, which is why I am writing this book in the first place.)

● **Coffee and tea** Try, in addition, not to drink too much coffee and/or tea. Both contain stimulants that increase anxiety and the stress reaction and caffeine has a direct stimulatory effect upon the heart. This is the last thing an overworked myocardium needs, when it is already trying to cope with the added driving force of extra adrenaline and noradrenaline. Decaffeinated coffee is far healthier and, because there is a rising demand for it, the market leader coffee brands are now being produced in a decaffeinated form. These are very palatable and are worth their small extra cost.

Herbal teas are also worth investigating if you have never tried them. Available from most health food shops and some supermarkets, the fruit and flower mixtures (apple, orange, passion fruit, rosehip and hibiscus flower) are as delicious as their ingredients suggest. Of special use in helping to induce a relaxed feeling are lemon balm and camomile teas.

● **Lack of exercise** Finally, among the 'don'ts' list is *'do not abandon exercise'*! Not only will it improve your overall physical fitness and stamina, it provides an ideal outlet for all your pent-up emotions arousing in you the primitive 'flight or fight' response. Take up jogging, swimming or dancing at home to your favourite records. This releases the stress, anger, pain, fear and resentment inside and reduces the risk of heart and arterial disease developing.

It also makes you *feel* much better. For one thing you get a sense of achievement, invaluable when you seem unable to cope adequately in certain other respects. For another, chemicals called endorphins are released from your brain cells in response to adequate amounts of aerobic exercise, say if you exercise for half an hour or longer and these have an anti-depressant effect, making you feel on top of the world.

Positive self-help

Relaxing sounds easy! So it is, if your inner feelings and your exterior surroundings are both conducive to it. You do not have to try – far less, to learn – to concentrate on 'letting go' when your thoughts are tranquil and untroubled and your body fit and well. At the end of a satisfying day of work and a delicious, unhurried evening meal, it is simplicity itself to switch on the television or the hi-fi and settle down in your armchair in front of the fire with a pleasant drink.

It is next to impossible to do so, though, on an evening when you arrive home after a trying journey to find that your central heating is not working, the cat has been sick on your new rug, you are inexplicably out of toilet paper and the shops are shut. Any dinner you do rustle up is most unlikely to reinstate that inner feeling of calmness and content we all covet and the temptation to retire to bed with the electric blanket on and an enormous whisky can be almost overwhelming!

One has, however, to *learn* to relax in circumstances that normally succeed in elevating one's blood pressure. This is the secret known and practised by those few people who really can cope with all that life throws at them, while retaining their patience and their sense of humour. *Deep breathing* is a simple action of incalculable benefit within this context. Relaxing one's *body muscles* is a necessary preliminary to relaxing mentally. Meditation is a superlative tool no one who practises it would ever be without.

Deep breathing

'Ordinary' deep breathing is simple to practise. Sit down or stand still, relax any muscles that are noticeably clenched, close your mouth and take in a deep breath through your nose, slowly filling your lungs to the count of six or seven. If you are a smoker or have recently given up tobacco, you will probably find that filling your lungs to capacity will bring on a tickly cough. If so, you will have to learn to breathe in just as far as you can comfortably tolerate. Hold your breath for five seconds and then breathe out slowly, again through your nose, to a count of five.

There are a number of physiological reasons why several breaths taken in this way are beneficial to the lungs, heart and autonomic nervous system – that part of your nervous system particularly closely involved in emotional and physical aspects of the stress response. Indian Yogis (Yoga experts) have a different explanation for the benefits of deep breathing and develop it into an art which they teach for the great benefits it can bestow on the whole body.

Learning Yoga as a means of learning to relax is a splendid idea. Ask your teacher, if you decide to join a group, to explain and demonstrate a variety of breathing techniques in addition to the usual asanas (Yoga positions.)

Relaxing your muscles

You can either lie down on the floor or bed when you do this or sit in a comfortable chair. Once you can eliminate feelings of physical tension, it is easier to develop a calm, tranquil mind. Starting with one foot and then the other, clench the muscles concerned (not so strongly that they start to cramp), then let go after five to ten seconds. Experience the loose, floppy feeling of the muscles when you have relaxed them, in contrast to the way they feel when constricted. This is how you should – and eventually will – feel all over!

Do the same with your left and then your right calf and thigh muscles, concentrating deeply upon each body area in turn and then work your way up your body, dealing in turn with the muscles of your buttocks, abdomen, back, shoulders (very important!), hands, lower and upper arms, neck, face and scalp (these can be mobilized slightly by frowning and then raising your eyebrows!)

Finally, screw your eyelids up tightly, grimace horribly, relax the muscles concerned and poke out your tongue – far enough to stretch it but not so far that you pull uncomfortably on the root. There is a saying that, if your tongue is really relaxed, the rest of you is bound to be relaxed too. Quickly recheck your muscle groups in case any have regained some of their usual tension and then close your eyes gently, taking three or four deep breaths as described above.

Meditating

You do not have to be religiously inclined or in any way unusual to benefit from meditating. How far you want to take the learning and practice of this art is up to you. Some Yoga teachers include meditation as part of their course and there are good books on the topic. Deep relaxation, combining a form of meditation, can also be learned on an individual basis from a hypnotherapist.

Here is a simple method you can try without further ado. Choose a time when you can extend deep breathing and muscular relaxation for a further 20 uninterrupted minutes. Do what you can to ensure this, by removing the telephone from the hook and selecting a room where you know you can be alone. Having relaxed all over, imagine yourself floating gently in a calm, warm sea, on a lilo or preferably just on your back, immersed in sun-warmed water. Experience the gentle lapping with your eyes closed and let your thoughts wander at random to the contemplation of pleasant relaxing things. (If you dislike water and the sea, picture yourself upon a delicate cloud of swansdown, being wafted softly, hither and thither by the gentlest and most refreshing of breezes.)

Then bring a pre-chosen image into your mind of a symbol you really love and feel at home with. I am presently using a rainbow – with those splendid, soft, ethereal colours no artist has ever *quite* captured and the strange magic of which rainbows are redolent, that of the mysterious 'crock of gold' at its end.

I can recommend this image as soothing and revitalizing. The crock of gold – there for everyone to find – is your 'light at the end of the tunnel', the freedom you *will* eventually know from present pain, misery and suffering. It is full of hope, beauty and love and the way to get the most value from it is to allow other thoughts to slide away, while you relax completely and picture your rainbow to the exclusion of all other images and thoughts. *See* it, in the full splendour of its natural beauty, and tell yourself that whenever you think of your rainbow (or whatever other image you prefer), instead of feeling uptight and stressed you will feel calm, capable and positive.

A little practice will make you perfect enough at the technique to derive untold psychological and physical benefits from it. Meditate, if you can, two or three times a week in a dimly-lit room with perhaps a candle or a joss stick burning, for 20 to 30 minutes at a time. Among its beneficial effects are a calming influence upon the central nervous system and the heart and it has been shown to have an excellent effect upon raised blood pressure and in patients suffering from angina.

Chapter 10

The extra protection from supplements

The simplest part of the Five-point Plan for a healthy heart is also one of the most important, and that is taking supplements of pure fish oil. These are best taken, as we saw earlier, as part of a total, structured programme, the constituents of which work side by side to reduce substantially the risk of cardiovascular disease. Backed by the other 'heart' nutrients, the essential fatty acid EPA can provide the optimal amount of 'Extra Protective Action' we all require.

A number of important breakthroughs have been made in the management of ischaemic heart and arterial disease in recent years. One of these, the fish oil supplement, is intended to be taken primarily for its protective action, although its curative function should not be overlooked. Its main role is to enable anyone who wishes to radically reduce the risks they run of suffering from ischaemic heart or arterial disease. At the same time it should also improve the condition of anyone who has already developed signs and symptoms of these conditions. For that reason, I will deal here with those research findings aimed at decreasing our cardiovascular disease risk factors rather than with specific treatments for acute illness likely to be carried out by doctors and other health professionals.

Vitamin E

This vitamin has been researched almost continuously for nearly half a century. Dr Evan Shute, a young obstetrician practising in Canada, first noticed that it helped prevent miscarriages in his patients. Later, he and his brother Wilfred investigated the effects of this vitamin more thoroughly and they pioneered its use in many medical conditions characterized by circulatory problems and faulty oxygenation.

The Shute Institute was established in 1946 in London, Ontario, and thousands of patients suffering from ischaemic heart disease have been helped by the use of vitamin E. It has beneficial effects upon the function of the blood cells, heart muscle strength and circulation, as well as helping to inhibit thrombosis. The oxygen-carrying capability of the blood is closely related to the vitamin E level and the rate of haemolysis – premature death of red blood cells – is one of the means for determining the vitamin E level in the body.

Dr Knut Haeger, of the Slottstaden Clinic in Malmo, Sweden, carried out a long-term study upon the use of vitamin E in the treatment of patients with moderately severe intermittent claudication, a disease which affects the arteries of the legs. Clogged by atheromatous plaques, the arteries supplying the lower limbs carry an inadequate supply of blood for the needs of the calf muscles. Patients experience severe pain after walking a certain distance (called their 'claudication distance') and are obliged to stop and rest until the pain passes away.

After an average of 18 month's trial, Dr Haeger reported a significant improvement in 73 per cent of the patients who received 100 iu of vitamin E three times a day. By comparison, only 19 per cent of the control group noticed significant improvement. He and his team concluded that, in conjunction with leg muscle exercises, vitamin E was a valuable addition to the therapy of this arterial disease.

The beneficial effects of vitamin E upon the circulation have been related to the fact that it reduces the stickiness of platelets and so helps to prevent the tendency to clump together and form clots. It also helps to reduce clotting by encouraging the formation of the anti-thrombotic prostaglandins and by inhibiting certain steps in the metabolism of vitamin E, which is normally responsible for promoting the beneficial clotting of blood.

Vitamin E supplements are recommended for patients with diseased coronary arteries and/or an increased tendency to thrombosis. The dosage is between 400 and 800 iu daily. Also Dr Hugh Sinclair found that an adequate intake of this vitamin was necessary for the optimal activity of the EPA he took in while on his Eskimo diet. I recommend taking 100 iu three times daily in order to acquire the cardioprotective action of this vitamin. In the case of patients taking anticoagulant therapy, it is a wise precaution to ask the advice of your doctor before taking vitamin E supplements regularly, as the latter can enhance the effects of such drugs.

Octacosanol

This fascinating substance is one of the active ingredients in wheatgerm oil. It is a fawn-coloured, waxy substance with the chemical structure of an alcohol and forms a protective coating on many varieties of plant leaf. It is thought to perform a wide variety of functions in nature and other sources of it, besides the kernel of wheat, include alfalfa, sugar cane and the cotton plant.

Forty years of research have shown that octacosanol has many valuable properties. It helps us resist the effects of stress, increases our vigour and physical endurance span, improves the function of muscle, including the myocardium and lowers systolic blood pressure. In helping us in times of stress, it both improves mental alertness and acuity, reaction time and reflex action *and*, at the same time, relaxes the muscles. In contrast to this, caffeine – to which we so often turn for its stimulatory action – has the unwanted effect of increasing our muscular tension. In addition, while octacosanol reduces blood pressure, caffeine elevates it. The secret of the different actions of these two substances is that while caffeine is an out-and-out stimulant, octacosanol is not. In fact, it relaxes both the muscle fibres and the autonomic nervous system, so that its overall effect is one of 'relaxed though increased alertness'. It also enables the body to maintain higher levels of activity for longer periods of time.

Not surprisingly, octacosanol is already of great interest to many sportsmen and women who wish to increase their physical endurance in a natural, drug-free way. It has been incorporated into at least one high energy tablet, alongside other energy-sustaining ingredients such as B complex vitamins, chromium, selenium, mineral transporters and desiccated liver. Apart from its action upon the heart muscle, I do recommend octacosanol as a useful supplement to anyone wanting to regain or maintain their state of physical fitness by daily aerobic exercise.

The well-known nutritional researchers Drs E. Cheraskin and W. M. Ringsdorf have this to say about octacosanol in their book *Psychodietetics* (Bantam Books):

> If you have been exercising regularly and eating properly, yet you are still having trouble reaching a high degree of physical fitness, the missing element may be octacosanol, a substance found in wheatgerm oil. After 20 years of research under controlled conditions with almost 1,000 people – middle-aged university faculty members, fraternity men, schoolboys, swimmers, wrestlers, track men – there is abundant evidence that octacosanol has beneficial effect on exercisers. It improves their *stamina* and *endurance*, *reduces heart stress* and *quickens reaction time*.

Further, two research scientists called Marinetti and Stolz

isolated a long-chain fatty alcohol from pig heart called 'cytochrome C reductase', an essential enzyme in the function of myocardial cells. It has been postulated that octacosanol might be involved in the fat fraction of this enzyme. This could be part of the explanation for octacosanol's ability to improve heart function.

A number of studies have shown that this substance benefited the T-wave of the electrocardiogram (ECG), the tracing cardiologists take of the electrical activity of heart muscle, from which a very great deal can be learned about the health or disease, the structure and function, of any particular patient's heart. The 'T-wave improvement' suggested an improved nutritional state of the myocardial heart muscle and a strengthening of the contractions measured electrically. Other studies have indicated that octacosanol aids the heart muscle in the retention of potassium, a mineral that is vital to the heart's function.

An additional bonus from taking octacosanol regularly is that it helps to reduce excess body fat. It does this in two ways: directly by increasing the metabolic rate, thereby increasing the rate at which we burn up food fuel for energy and indirectly by calming the nerves, thereby decreasing any tendency to eat as a response to stress and tension. Weight reduction is of great importance, as we have seen, to the maintenance of a healthy heart and circulation and to the practice of regular exercise.

Various suggestions have been made about the optimal quantity of octacosanol to be taken daily as a nutritional supplement. In *The Alternative Dictionary of Symptoms and Cures* (Century Hutchinson, 1986), I suggest a dose of 6,000 mcg daily when it is being used to treat established coronary artery disease. However, a dose as low as 1,000 mcg daily can prove beneficial to healthy people wanting extra protection against cardiovascular risk factors.

Carnitine

Proteins are composed of building units named amino acids and it is into these structural components that the protein in our diet is broken down during the process of digestion. Carnitine is an amino acid and, in common with other amino acids, it has specific biochemical roles to play in human metabolism. Its main function is to transport fatty acids into the mitochondria – these are the 'power houses' of our tissue cells within which both fatty acids and glucose combine with oxygen to generate energy.

Myocardial muscle contains a high level of carnitine, one of the reasons being its dependence upon long-chain fatty acids as a source of energy (it utilizes them for between 48 and 70 per cent of its total energy requirements). These energy requirements, as we saw earlier in the book, are considerable, since, on average, the heart contracts 70 to 80 times per minute, every single minute we are alive. Over a 24-hour period it pumps the equivalent of 8,183l (1,800 gallons) of blood through the 20,675km (75,000 miles) of blood vessels that our bodies contain.

A number of medical trials have indicated the probable protective action carnitine can afford the myocardium in people whose coronary arteries are clogged – or partially clogged – with atheromatous plaque. In a recent study, this amino acid was administered intravenously to patients with ischaemic heart disease and their myocardia were found both to utilize fatty acids more efficiently and to accumulate less lactate during prescribed exercise. This meant that their tolerance of exercise had improved. Improved mental alertness has also been noted in patients taking carnitine and people suffering from intermittent claudication have shown improved muscle function.

Leon Chaitow, the world-renowned nutritional expert, commented on a report of the above trial that carnitine can be recommended as 'part of the safe, first-aid type measure employed by nutritionally orientated practitioners in conditions involving myocardial distress.'

As a doctor, I also recommend carnitine as a common-sense addition to daily supplements aimed at affording extra protection against cardiovascular disease. A suitable dose for most adults is 200 mg three times daily, increasing after a week to 400 mg three times daily.

Taurine and histidine

The amino acid taurine has been used successfully in the treatment of congestive heart failure. In this condition, the heart is working inadequately and pressure builds up within the circulatory system, causing congestion of the lungs (hence the condition's name) and oedema (swelling, generally in the feet and lower legs, due to the accumulation of tissue fluid). Rheumatic heart disease, that is, damage to the heart valves secondary to rheumatic fever, is one cause of congestive heart failure.

A group of 58 patients with this condition were studied in a controlled medical trial. Over a 28-day period, each patient received either a 'dummy' placebo tablet or 6 grams of taurine daily in three divided doses. The symptoms of breathlessness (which is a cardinal sign in congestive heart failure), oedema and heart palpitations improved significantly, in the patients receiving taurine. And improvements were also noted in chest X-rays and in the overall function of the patients concerned.

Taurine was effective in these ways, whether or not the patients were receiving digitalis for their heart condition. No significant improvement occurred in patients who had received the placebo instead of taurine. It has also been found to encourage cholesterol to stay in solution in the blood in its lipoprotein form, in preference to coming out of solution within the walls of arteries to form plaques.

Because of the beneficial effects taurine has been shown to have in patients with cardiac disease, I recommend patients who are especially at risk (those with signs of already existing coronary artery disease) to take it in supplement form. A usual dose for an adult is 500 mg to 1 gram daily.

Histidine, another amino acid, improves the circulation of the blood within the coronary arteries and is able to lower the blood pressure by causing blood vessel walls to relax.

In addition to these special supplements, a natural (non-synthetic) multivitamin supplement should be taken daily, as well as a multimineral one in chelated form (this is the form in which minerals are most easily absorbed by the body). One gram of vitamin C (a major anti-stress vitamin, together with naturally occurring bioflavonoids) and a vitamin E complex supplement should also be added.

Pure fish oil supplement

Adding a pure fish oil supplement to your daily diet is the most important step you can take in minimizing your risk of developing cardiovascular disease. The trials of fish oil supplements quoted earlier were performed using MaxEPA which is now available on prescription. It is mainly used in treating patients with established heart and coronary artery disease.

Both MaxEPA and other pure fish oils are produced from the flesh of oily fish. The liver is not used, because of its high concentration of vitamin A.

The best way to get into the habit of taking your daily protective supplements is by taking them with a drink, after a meal, at the same time each day. Even if you have a fish meal, still take your supplements. The EPA contained in fresh fish and the fish oil supplement is entirely natural and completely free of harmful effects.

Glossary

Alpha-linolenic acid: Essential fatty acid needed for manufacture of heart-protecting EPA.

Angina: Chest pain, sometimes extending into neck and down arms, due to reduced blood supply to heart muscle.

Arachidonic acid: The 'mixed blessing' essential fatty acid, giving rise to both protective and harmful prostaglandins.

Artery: Thick, muscular blood vessel carrying oxygen-rich blood from heart to body tissues and organs.

Atheroma: Fatty material deposited as plaques (plates) in the walls of arteries, eventually clogging them.

Atherosclerosis: Arterial disease due to atheroma.

Bleeding time: Time taken for blood to clot, sealing an injured area.

Blood pressure: Expressed in millimetres of mercury as two figures e.g. 130/85. The upper figure (systolic) is the pressure of the blood on the walls of the arteries, the lower (diastolic) is the resistance afforded by the small vessels (arterioles) to blood entering them.

Cholesterol: Natural fat needed by the body but contributing to atherosclerosis (and therefore heart disease) when present in excess.

Cis-linoleic acid: Essential fatty acid giving rise to

protective prostaglandins and (occasionally) arachidonic acid.

Claudication: Cramping pain in calf muscles triggered by exercise and caused by narrowing of arteries to the legs.

Coronary thrombosis: Heart attack due to blood clot (thrombus) blocking coronary artery supplying blood to the heart.

DHA: Essential fatty acid present in fish oil vital to brain, nerve and eye tissue.

ECG (electrocardiogram): Tracing on paper of electrical activity of heart muscle, used to diagnose heart conditions.

EPA: Essential fatty acid found in fish oil, providing protection against thrombosis, and arterial and heart disease.

Essential fatty acids (EFAS): Polyunsaturated fatty acids required for cellular health, and for the manufacture of prostaglandins.

Free radicals: Unstable, highly-charged molecular fragments which, when present in excess, encourage tissue degeneration and atheroma formation.

HDL cholesterol: Useful cholesterol helping to keep arteries healthy.

Heart attack: Damage (fatal or otherwise) to heart muscle resulting from lack of blood supply. Causes include acute spasm or blockage by a bloodclot of diseased coronary arteries. (*See also* **Myocardial infarction**).

Ischaemia: Deficient blood supply to a tissue or organ.

Ischaemic heart disease (IHD): Heart disease, angina, etc., due to ischaemia.

LDL cholesterol: Injurious cholesterol promoting atheroma formation and arterial disease.

Lipoprotein: Combination of lipids and protein, in which lipids (body fats) are transported in the bloodstream.

Monounsaturated fat: Dietary fat, chemically halfway between saturated and polyunsaturated varieties, offering some protection against arterial and heart disease, e.g. olive oil.

Myocardial infarction (MI): Death of an area of heart muscle or myocardium, due to lack of blood supply.

Platelets: Minute, cell-like bodies in bloodstream that promote clotting.

Polyunsaturated fatty acids (PUFAs): Healthy dietary fats derived from plant and seed oils and oily fish, giving rise in body to prostaglandins.

Red blood cell: Chief cell in bloodstream, and transports oxygen from lungs to rest of body.

Saturated fat: Animal fats found in red meat, dairy products, etc., which in excess encourages the formation of atheroma and arterial/heart disease.

Saturation (chemical): The addition of as much hydrogen to the carbon chain in a fatty acid as it is capable of absorbing.

Stroke: Sudden damage to area of brain tissue due to a blocked artery or burst blood vessel (cerebral haemorrhage).

Thrombosis: Abnormal clotting of blood within a blood vessel.

Vein: Thin-walled blood vessel transporting oxygen-poor blood back from tissues and organs to heart and lungs.

Ventricular fibrillation (VF): Grave disturbance of heart's regular pumping action, in which its lower chambers or ventricles contract haphazardly and without useful effect.

White blood cells: Second most numerous cell in bloodstream, involved in fighting infection and promoting inflammation to deal with foreign material.

Index

Fish Oil